Live your best life!

Live your best life!

Whole Mind, Whole Body, Complete Health
The integrated guide to diet,
happiness and life

Dr Lily Tomas and Greg de Jong

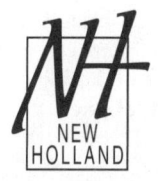

NEW HOLLAND

First published in Australia in 2008 by
New Holland Publishers (Australia) Pty Ltd
Sydney • Auckland • London • Cape Town

1/66 Gibbes Street Chatswood NSW 2067 Australia
218 Lake Road Northcote Auckland New Zealand
86 Edgware Road London W2 2EA United Kingdom
80 McKenzie Street Cape Town 8001 South Africa

Copyright © 2008 in text: Lily Tomas and Greg de Jong
Copyright © 2008 New Holland Publishers (Australia) Pty Ltd

All rights reserved. No part of this publication may be reproduced, stored in a retrieval system or transmitted, in any form or by any means, electronic, mechanical, photocopying, recording or otherwise, without the prior written permission of the publishers and copyright holders.

National Library of Australia Cataloguing-in-Publication Data:

Tomas, Lily.

Live your best life! : whole mind, whole body, complete health, the integrated guide to nutrition, happiness and life / authors, Dr Lily Tomas ; Greg de Jong.

ISBN: 9781741106206 (pbk.)

Nutrition. Diet. Health self-care. Stress management.

De Jong, Greg.
613.7

Publisher: Fiona Schultz
Managing Editor: Lliane Clarke
Designer: Simon Rattray
Cover Design: Natasha Hayles
Production Assistant: Liz Malcolm
Printer: McPherson's Printing Group

10 9 8 7 6 5 4 3 2 1

Although every effort has been made to verify the accuracy of the information contained in this book, it must not be treated as a substitute for medical or professional opinion or advice. Neither the author nor the publishers can be held responsible for any loss, injury or inconvenience sustained by any person arising out of the use, or misuse, of the suggestions, or the failure to take medical care.

Inside

Preface: Be Happy 7

Section 1: It's Simple, So Smile! **10**
1: Towards a Happy Mindbody 11
2: Keep It Simple 13
3: The Pleasure Principle 14
4: So Why Aren't You Exercising? 17
5: Why Will You Change? 21
6: Riding the Rollercoaster 24

Section 2: Changing Your Life from Head to Toe **28**
1: Loving Your Self, Loving Life 29
2: Emotions, Reason, Action 33
3: Building Better Relationships 42
4: Living with Passion 48
5: Towards Stress-less Living 51
6: To Laugh, To Sing, To Dance, To Make Love 60
7: Learning to Be 64
8: Goodnight, Sweetheart 66

Section 3: Forget Dieting, Simply Choose Healthy Eating **69**
1: Understanding Your Hunger 70
2: A Quick Look at Energy Balance 76
3: Understanding What You Eat 80
4: Creating a Healthy Plate 92
5: Enjoying Your Healthy Eating Plan 100
6: The Quest for Magical Foods 114
7: Understanding Food Intolerances 121
8: The Food Elimination Regime 126
9: Eat Out and Enjoy 135
10: Drink and Be Merry 139
11: So What About Your Weight? 141
12: The Recipe-less Recipe Guide 143

Section 4: Examining the Health and Treatment Continuum **146**
1: Health, Dysfunction, Disease: When Should You Intervene? 147
2: Can Food Be Thy Medicine? 155
3: To Supplement or Not To Supplement? 165
4: The Place of Medicine 184

Section 5: Investigating Your Personal Supplement Needs **192**
1: Cellular Health 194
2: Gastrointestinal Health 205
3: Demystifying the Liver 215
4: Cardiovascular Health 226
5: Respiratory and Airways Health 236
6: Insulin Resistance, Diabetes and Weight Loss 242
7: Hormone Health 252
8: Neurotransmitter Health 270
9: Bones, Joints and Muscles 280
10: Creating a Healthy Immune System 288
11: Vision, Hearing and Headaches 299
12: Skin, Nails and Hair 302
13: Anti-Ageing 306

Section 6: Putting It All Together **309**
1: Getting Happy! 310
2: Individualising Your Personal Health 315
3: Addressing Primary Health Dysfunctions 316
4: Addressing Other Health Dysfunctions 319
5: Weaning Supplementation 320
6: Health Maintenance 323
7: Health and Food Intolerance Reviews 324

Appendix: Finding a Professional 326

PREFACE

Be Happy

The one thing in life that we all really want is simply to be happy.
 To be at peace with ourselves and with the surrounding world.
 To be content, to be fulfilled, to be free from worries.
 Simply to be free.
 When we are happy, we are healthy, in the true sense of the word. Conversely, when we are not happy, we are not healthy. We may, for example, take every vitamin and mineral supplement under the sun in order to heal ourselves, yet we can never attain true health if we are only healthy on the physical level. We must be healthy in whole, not in part.
 Put simply, this includes a healthy Body, a healthy Mind and a healthy Spirit. This is true, no matter which way you perceive life, whether you are spiritual, religious, agnostic or atheist. Your Spirit is your essential essence of Being, your drive, your will. It is that strong will to survive that may only become truly known to yourself at dire times if, or when, it is needed.
 There is an old Chinese proverb:

When there is happiness in the heart,
there is happiness in the home.
When there is happiness in the home,
there is happiness in the nation.
When there is happiness in the nation,
there is happiness in the world.

Science has now virtually proven this in the realm of quantum physics. There is no doubt that the way we think affects not only the way we behave, but also the way others behave. It has been shown time and time again that, as mere observers to events occurring outside ourselves, our thoughts are able to profoundly influence such events.

There are now fields of combined quantum physics and medicine that have emerged which explain these elaborate and intricate connections beautifully. Such fields are beyond the scope of this particular book , but it's a comforting thought to know they are out there.

The recently emerged medical fields of psychoneuroimmunology and psychoneuroendocrinology explain what is currently known of the amazing connection between our mind and brain hormones (our neurotransmitters), the health of our gut, our thyroid and reproductive hormones and our immune system. For example, we are now aware that serotonin (one of our happy brain neurotransmitters) is not only produced in our brain, but also in our digestive system.

This not only adds new meaning to the saying 'You are what you eat', but also points to the fact that what you eat can profoundly affect how happy you feel, and, indeed, how clearly you think.

Our body is in a constant state of change. We are dynamic beings, our molecules constantly in motion. We are never static. This is why no matter how healthy we think we are at any given moment, we always have the potential to turn the tide towards a healthier (or unhealthier) destiny.

The way our life falls is therefore ultimately influenced by how we think and how we feel. It is important to note that this does not mean that we create our own illnesses, but we certainly do have an incredible influence. It really is no coincidence that the word "disease" is derived simply from dis-ease. We as individuals therefore have more control than we realise in alleviating or influencing our feelings of dis-ease.

The simple concept to understand from the first is that happiness is vital to our health on so many levels. We must do everything we can to achieve happiness in our lives.

The aim of this book is therefore to touch on important principles common to each and every one of us. It is not our intention to spend too long on any one particular area, specific disease state or subgroup of people. Rather, it is our intention to keep our message as simple as we can, while providing you with effective, applicable and practical information.

We begin with the anonymous words of someone wise whom we respectfully acknowledge:

'Live it, Let it, Love it, Let it go.'

Important Note

This book proceeds from the simple to the sexy. Sexy is wine and chocolates, nights out at the cinema, fast cars and, for the authors of this book who deal primarily in total health care, the use of simple nutritional supplement regimes which bring about amazing changes in people's lives. Perhaps we need to get out more?!

Yet the simple cannot be overlooked when it comes to chasing the prize of optimal health. Many medical professionals find laser surgery, high tech drugs and the latest computer imaging sexy, but you need to go a long way down the road of ill health to fulfil these desires. Satisfying for them, but not necessarily for you!

If you want to feel sexy, vibrant, passionate, 110% alive, you cannot bypass the simple. While we have no doubt that the nutritional supplement programs presented in the latter part of this book will further progress your health journey, the first three sections are dedicated to the fundamental principles of healthy living; Self Fulfilment, Emotional Intelligence, Exercise and Diet.

YOU MUST READ THE SECTIONS 1 TO 3 FIRST. SIMPLE HEALTH PRINCIPLES CANNOT BE BYPASSED OR SUBSTITUTED. THEY ARE FUNDAMENTALLY NECESSARY AS THE FOUNDATION TO ANY FURTHER HEALTH ADVICE.

With persistence and dedication, the principles and programs in this book are bound to alter your life. What you do when you get to 110% sexy is all up to you!

SECTION 1

It's Simple, So Smile!

Few, if any, attempts at lifestyle modification will succeed if overly complicated. Yet ironically, that is what many of us seek: complicated approaches that require professional interventions rather than simple life solutions. Many of us are drawn to scientific theories argued as fact, or magical formulas or recipes that need to be followed. One wonders how our ancestors survived without the many textbooks we now drive ourselves to read in the name of 'Self Help'.

We therefore write the majority of the first half of this book from a place of justifying what otherwise is common knowledge and common sense. We give you permission to explore simple health rules such as, 'Make yourself happy in some way, every day', 'Go for a walk once a day', 'Get a good night's sleep' and 'Eat a variety of natural foods in moderation'.

This is our primary focus, particularly in this section. To keep it simple. To keep your focus on what really matters; that life should be a pleasurable experience. Sexy, if you like. Sexy is good because it gets your attention, but it also indicates that life should be lived with pleasure and a moderate and healthy degree of indulgence, whoever we are, whatever our weight, our income, or our position on the work or social scale.

Our aim is to encourage you **Simply to Be Happy with Simply Being**.

1

Towards a Happy Mindbody

It is an indisputable fact that unless you have a serious and presently active medical disorder you are 90 per cent in control of your health 99.9 per cent of the time.

Not through the use of prescription drugs and modern medical science.

Nor homeopathy, herbal remedies or other forms of healing. Good health is available through the simple choices you make about what your Mindbody consumes, experiences and expresses in your interaction with the natural world in which you live.

In specific terms this means:

- Acknowledging your own power in choosing to be happy rather than hurt
- Making sensible and balanced food choices
- Participating in moderate physical exercise
- Learning to relax and enjoy life
- Achieving a good night's sleep
- Surrounding yourself with a healthy environment
- Living life with passion across all levels; physically, intellectually, emotionally and spiritually

AND

- ... if you need to take prescription medication, taking it sensibly and to your doctor's recommendations.

These are the fundamental constituents of healthy living. Furthermore, they are also the fundamentals of happy living.

For the truth of the matter is, people rarely fall ill as if by fatalistic design. Although we may be predisposed to disease by our genetic inheritance, it is rarely the case that our genes enforce disease upon us with 100% certainty. Nor is it true that we are unable to moderate the level of disease manifesting in our bodies simply through healthy living.

Rather our actions and behaviours mediate whether or not we inherit the healthy or unhealthy influences within our predestined genetic code.

Ignore this truth at your peril.

For if ignorance is your choice, you are destined for a life dependent on medical practitioners, conventional or otherwise, accepting the gradual decay of your life into chronic disease as if predestined by God or chance, however you wish to interpret it.

But life within your Mindbody need not be so.

It can be lived with vibrant energy, purpose and passionate self-fulfilment.

This is the choice we are presenting to you in this book. To take command of a happy Mindbodyspirit and live life by a set of healthy principles, in order to regain optimal wellbeing.

2

Keep It Simple

Are you aware that 30 minutes of brisk walking per day is all you need to get most of what you want out of exercise? That committing yourself to simple eating guidelines can direct you towards a life of health, vitality and happiness far more than any complex fad diet? And that avoiding the need for long lists of medical drugs by simple preventative health steps such as these can minimise the risk of many prescription related complications?

Remember that the key ingredient is You, that the authority on what is right and what is wrong is your own, and that the truth of the outcome is for you alone to decide, based upon how you feel; physically, mentally, emotionally, spiritually.

So here is the first key step:

Keep it simple!

Do not believe for one moment that the more complicated you try and make your diet, exercise program or other health regime, the better life will necessarily become. If so, you are going to make a lot of doctors, naturopaths, physiotherapists and other medical practitioners happy with your health dollar. Each of these practitioners have a place, but only after you have started on a simple course towards health and happiness as outlined in this book.

Complicate matters if you must, but only after getting the fundamentals right, and only if you enjoy the increased complexity of any program you set yourself.

Otherwise, keep it simple, pleasurable, sexy ...

3

The Pleasure Principle

Here is your first simple health intervention.

Every day

I will find a way

To make myself happy!

How are you going to achieve this? Start by circling any of the following that you would enjoy doing today:

Reading ☺ Going to a Movie ☺ Listening to Music ☺ Painting ☺ Writing a Letter to a Friend ☺ Playing with a Pet ☺ Playing a Computer Game ☺ Playing with your Child/ren ☺ Sewing ☺ Singing ☺ Sculpting ☺ Cooking ☺ Taking a Bath ☺ Having a Laugh ☺ Getting a Massage ☺ Meditating ☺ Burning some Aromatherapy Candles ☺ Gardening ☺ Tennis ☺ Football ☺ Basketball ☺ Golf ☺ Daydreaming ☺ Walking in the Park, the Bush or at the Beach ☺ Enjoying the Intimate Company of a Partner ☺ Watching a Comedy ☺ Playing a Musical Instrument ☺ Enjoying a Quality Eating Treat ☺ Taking in a Play ☺ Writing a Poem, a Novel or a Song ☺ Redecorating, Shopping or Pottering in the Garden ☺ Planning a Dream Holiday whether going there or not ☺ Becoming a Collector ☺ Going Fishing ☺ Sunbaking ☺ Driving ☺ Going to a Gallery, Museum or Zoo ☺ Photo Taking ☺ Relaxing in a Sauna or Spa ☺ Enjoying Darts, Snooker, or a Beer at the Pub ☺ It's Pleasure Time, give your shoulders a rub!

Let's begin with an obvious truth almost universally forgotten by anyone preoccupied with the intricate details of their diet, exercise program or counselling sessions.

If you're not happy with your life, your chance of committing to any long-term health program is highly questionable.

For if you're not that inspired by exercise but realise you simply have to do it, you will need to be happy in the rest of your life first in order to maintain this commitment to yourself. Otherwise, you're simply going to say, 'Why bother?'

When you need to make the next simple choice between the fast food drive-through and making a healthy lunch at home you'll simply say, 'Why wait?' More to the point, you'll probably dive in for the high-carbohydrate lunch hoping for the sugar kick to set you free from your current low.

But if you're feeling good about life, or at least your present moment in life, then chances are you're going to say, 'I want to eat well, I want to exercise, so I can enjoy my life even more'. So you'll make the extra effort to walk the extra mile and take the extra time to make your salad bowl.

The reality is, as many of you may already be arguing, that bringing your whole life to a happy state is not always going to be easy. You may have major issues to resolve, relationship crises, financial pressures, stressful circumstances ... the list of life's difficulties can be long. Yet your next mood state, your next moment of living, does not need to be tied to your ongoing life stress. It can be an individual moment of motivational pleasure.

The Pleasure Principle involves developing the skill of being able to live in the moment.

Look at the list of activities at the start of this chapter. Given a general level of health, not one of these activities is dependent upon any ongoing life situation for you to participate. Each and every pleasure activity can be undertaken regardless of relationship crisis, financial pressure or stressful circumstance, if you choose to make time for the Pleasure Principle.

Here's the first practical suggestion to apply to your life. It's not diet, it's not exercise and it's not a list of supplements or medications.

It is as simple as this:

Set aside a minimum of 30 minutes per day to pleasure your Self regardless of anyone else's needs.

No excuses. You are going to learn to be Self-First. This is an important concept to understand. Being Self-First is not being Selfish. Being Selfish means you do not care about others. Being Self-First simply allows you to gain and maintain the energy and vitality you need to be able to be there for others when you are needed.

You simply can't give fully to anybody else over the long-term without becoming physically and emotionally drained unless you are fulfilled in your Self first. Many of you have probably experienced this and know in your heart that it is true.

Life needs to be pleasurable to be motivating, and the single motivation that can be guaranteed is the pleasure of living for the daily fruits of life that can be experienced independent of greater life drama.

Please do not take this suggestion lightly. Write your own list of activities that will make you happy and pin it to the fridge. You may particularly need this list to break through low or stressful periods of life when you may in fact need to force yourself to take time out and commit to making yourself happy!

If you are unable to do this yourself, then we strongly recommend you seek professional help now in order to achieve this most basic of healthy life principles. Because if you cannot create moments of happiness in your life, it is likely that you are depressed and in need of assistance.

4

So Why Aren't You Exercising?

We live in the age of information in which to deny that you have not heard basic health messages pronounced through all forms of media would be difficult, if not a lie. And while there may be an acceptable level of confusion over the diet dilemma with such a multitude of diets to choose from, the same cannot be said for exercise. All of us should be aware that to retain a suitable level of cardiovascular fitness, we need to be doing a minimum of three to five exercise sessions a week. This can be as simple as a brisk walk on the spot.

If you are already achieving this, congratulations.

If not, then what excuses are you coming up with to justify ignoring this most basic and indisputable health necessity?

The reality is, short of physical incapacity, there are few if any reasons that acceptably justify not being able to achieve this level of exercise. That is, if you value your health highly enough. Here are a few excuses you may presently be using:

'I have no time.'
'I don't like sport.'
'I need to look after the children.'
'I'm in poor health.'
'I can't afford equipment.'
'I don't have the energy.'
'I don't have transport to get to a place where I can exercise.'
'I'm too fat.'
'I'm too shy or afraid to go outdoors.'
'It's raining.'
'Exercise is boring.'
'I'm lazy.'

A lot of excuses, aren't there? But they can all be dispelled, and the few that might not be so easily dispelled—usually medical issues—can often be worked around with a little more thought (for example, using a seated or reclining bicycle, doing bed and chair exercises, using a therapy pool etc.).

Exercise is only one area where our excuses can seem lame on closer examination; the same holds true for most of the lifestyle issues examined in this book.

The truth of the matter is, when it comes to simple health principles, 90 per cent of your excuses have been created to justify inaction. Because it is often far easier to take a moment to think up suitable excuses for not acting, as compared to the effort required to exercise, seek healthy food solutions or even lie down to do nothing more than relax!

So how do you counter the power of excuses and the procrastination that results?

The first step is to make yourself aware of the reasoning behind your excuses in the first place. The second step is to prevent yourself from taking up any course of inaction that prevents your pursuit of healthy living. This will depend largely on your level of motivation, which we shall discuss further in the next chapter. In other words, you need to become aware of when you are making excuses, and not allow yourself to succumb to them.

You might be saying, well aren't some reasons acceptable? Well, yes, on individual occasions. But after you have used most excuses once you can learn to prepare for them in the future so as not to make them justifiable a second time.

Do you actually have to fall into the use of an excuse before you can provide for a way of no longer justifying it?

Not if you put a little forethought into any particular health plan and work out what may be your likely problems and excuses to begin with. Then counter the excuse with a plan that reduces potential roadblocks in the future.

And if you have a reasonable excuse that limits your action today?

So be it. Accept your day's limitation and make pleasurable, or at least practical, use of your time. Guilt is a useless emotion anyway unless you can act to change it into something positive. Definitely do not chastise yourself and pull yourself down into a state where you no longer think you can commit to your health plan.

After all, throwing out a health plan completely because you weren't 100 per cent compliant is going to do you far less good than a health plan followed 90 per cent, 80 per cent, or even 50 per cent of the time.

Easy Does It Exercise

Here are your fundamental rules in order to achieve 90 per cent of the health rewards from exercise. Which of course include decreased risk of cardiovascular disease, reduced risk of Metabolic Syndrome and Type 2 Diabetes Mellitus and decreased risk of mental health conditions, to name only a few.

1. Exercise for 30 minutes
2. At least five days per week
3. At a level that makes you puff, but not so hard that you are breathless
4. Perform any activity or exercise that brings you to a level of a puff for 30 minutes

And in case you are unfit enough that 30 minutes is out of the question, the health authorities even give you a probation period to get there...

5. If required you can break up your 30 minutes into several exercise sessions, as long as they are greater than five minute intervals.

Options are swimming, cycling, gym sessions, stair climbing, jogging, power walking or callisthenics. But they also might include any sport of your choosing, as well as bushwalking, playing with your kids, wrestling your dog, social dancing, sailing, windsurfing, rock climbing, dancing naked in your bedroom, dancing naked with your partner in the bedroom ...

So there are always options. If you have any doubts, talk to an exercise therapist, physiotherapist, chiropractor, osteopath, doctor or other health professional you trust on this matter.

Here are some added benefits you can obtain from exercise, and what activities to do in order to achieve these benefits.

1. **Flexibility** is important for preventing injuries. You should start any intense exercise session with warm-up stretches. A more focused approach to flexibility can be achieved through *yoga*, as long as care is taken in approaching some of the more challenging positions. A qualified instructor is strongly recommended here.
2. **Strength** training allows you to build muscle bulk and tone. Interestingly, increased muscle bulk has been associated with increased longevity, so if you want to live longer, take up resistance training. A balanced *gym* or *home weight program* incorporating all of the body's major muscle groups at least twice per week is what you will need.
3. **Balance** is also a very important factor in healthy ageing, particularly for post-menopausal women at risk of fractures due to the combination of osteoporosis and falls. *Tai Chi* has been proven to increase balance in healthy older people, subsequently diminishing the risk of falls and fractures.
4. **Core Stability** is a method of training the back and abdominal muscles to protect the lower back region. Since lower back pain is prevalent in the general population, it is sensible to understand how to strengthen this region effectively. *Pilates* or *Swiss Ball Classes* generally focus on teaching core stability.

5

Why Will You Change?

The key to any sustained change is to remain motivated. It is no coincidence that the word 'motivation' comes from the same root word as 'emotion'. For both terms derive from the act of movement.

And what moves you to act?

The answer is **E-MOTION**.

For our emotions are the impulse and inner drive that guide our actions, while a lack of emotion, or in some instances overwhelming negative emotions, such as fear or depression, lead to inertia, procrastination and inaction.

Therefore, to motivate yourself you will need an impassioned reason empowering your intent to change.

Objective reasoning may justify an action, but if there is no true passion behind the action, there is little chance of sustained commitment into the future. Your best chance at successful change therefore is to be passionate about your intent by building emotive arguments engaging you to act.

Healthy impassioned reasoning can be motivated by two sources:
1) In an effort to move away from negative emotions; hurt, fear, loneliness, guilt, shame and so forth (and in the specific case of health related motivations; pain, fatigue, discomfort, anxiety, depression or any other physical or emotional sign or symptom of disease or ill health).
2) Or as an effort to move towards positive emotions; victory, love, intimacy, connection, happiness, energy, wellbeing, vitality and so on.

To empower yourself with motivation, it is necessary to investigate your reasoning and seek as many passionate arguments directing you towards desired change as possible. Make a list. Be thorough. Be passionate. And every morning take a moment's reflection to re-empower yourself with the reasons motivating you towards healthy change. The list might look something like this:

- Feeling good, feeling great
- Being happy
- Being less hurt
- Looking better
- Fitting into a new wardrobe.

Make the list as long as you like, providing the arguments are healthy and personally meaningful. Create signs and place them around the house. It's amazing how effective subliminal messages can be. You'll probably only need one list for most of the suggestions in this book, for in reality they all build towards the same goal : less hurtful, more gainful Mindbody states.

What if you feel you are coming up short on the motivation side? Perhaps you started off empowered but feel your drive flattening a little with time.

Then keep creating powerful and passionate motivations of your own.

Set yourself empowering reward bonuses for achieving health milestones.

'I commit myself to changing my life, my relationships, my emotional intelligence, and in three months' time I'm taking my partner on a fun-filled holiday (kids can stay with grandma!).'

'At 12 weeks of committed regular exercise I'm taking myself on a white water rafting trip!'

'If I continue my Healthy Eating Plan for another six weeks, I'm having myself an indulgence day with my friends and don't spare the chocolate!'

Remember, there are three simple rules to motivate your Self:
1. If it takes me away from personal pain (discomfort, disease), I will do it.
2. It if takes me towards personal gain (energy, vitality, happiness), I will do it.
3. I will reward myself for the commitments I have made, regardless, because I am worth it.

Whenever you doubt your ability to commit to a health change, list your motivations.

And keep listing them until you feel motivated to act.

Write your first list **NOW**.

6

Riding the Roller Coaster

Most health commitments last a week. Many commitments last two weeks. Some commitments last three weeks ... and then the drift sets in.

Be it a diet, exercise program or commitment to relaxation, the longer the road, the greater the likelihood of facing a stumbling block.

But when you get knocked down, do you get up again?

Or are you down for the count?

If you have fully investigated your motivations and potential excuses you have a head start on beating the breakdown blues. But only a start. There are a few more qualities you may need to rely on to ride the roller coaster of any Life Plan.

And these include:

Patience

Everyone wants to see change. But the reality of attempting health change often comes down to this: if it happens too fast, it does not last. There are both physiological and psychological reasons for this. Patience and perseverance entrench change without shocking the Mindbody. Conversely, rapidly attacking the Mindbody with a new health plan replicates a stressful crisis rather than a sustainable health intervention.

And what will your body do once the 'crisis' is over? Reject the new living plan and pack back on what the Mindbody considers to be the protective pounds.

Patience isn't the easiest quality to learn. We all want to feel better, healthier, happier, NOW. And we often give up when it doesn't happen fast enough. So in order to support patience, consider realistic goals.

'No marathon next week but maybe in six months'.
'Half a kilogram a week means ideal body weight in one year.'
'Coping with a relationship crisis now, growing back to where we were week by week, month by month.'

These are patient goals, goals you can live with, cope with and sustain without adding more stress and pressure to your already pressured life.

Persistence

With patience comes persistence. There are going to be mistakes, let-downs, temptations (and what would life be without temptations?). But the key is to persist with the majority of what you know is right. And enjoy the shortfalls that come your way. For if you really have entrenched your desire for health change within impassioned motivation, while restricting your excuses through reasoned awareness, then any shortfalls are more likely to be spontaneous and joyous opportunities.

The greatest risk to persistence is perfectionism.

Be aware of beliefs dictating that life should take the ideal route and if it does not then it isn't worth pursuing. 100 per cent health perfection would be wonderful, but so too would 75 per cent health perfection if you are doing nothing (0 per cent!) right now. Persist with what you can and motivate yourself to better this, but realise a single small step forward is better than any number of steps back!

Positive Attitude

Here is a vital component to a healthy Mindbody. Be positive. Be proactive. Pursue life with optimism. Wherever possible live life as if all is going to fall your way. Make a commitment to recite affirmations that encourage your own personal growth and destiny, such as:

'I am destined for happiness, health and a life extraordinary.'
'I am creating my own destiny.'
'As I intend, I manifest.'

Or whatever catchphrase most inspires you. Find ways to visualise your goals. Or choose music that fills you with inspirational feelings. Dress for success. Create your own environment of positive living.

For with a positive attitude comes self-belief, an understanding that you can achieve the goals that you have set for yourself. And a smile. For a smile can change your world if you feel it thoroughly enough through your entire being.

So make your smile the test of your body image. Not your weight, your present appearance, whether you have a partner or not.

The eyes may be the window to your soul, but your smile is your soul's joyous expression of its positive affirmation for living.

So live life with a smile, being positive in all that you do and aspire to do.

Personalised Achievement

How you benchmark your day to day or ultimate achievements is really up to you. You should not dance to anyone else's drum, idealistic images or dictates. Life is about what you want it to be, and if anyone tries to convince you otherwise, either by direct argument, surreptitious or even subconscious endeavour, just smile and acknowledge that they are on their own separate life path with their own life challenges and lessons to learn.

Don't give away your personal power to govern your own destiny for this is indeed your birthright.

So it is time to get personal with your goal setting.

What do **YOU** want of **YOUR** health and **YOUR** happiness?

Your answer does not need be a perfect ideal. It only needs to be **YOUR** answer. As long as you accept your own consequences, so be it. If you enjoy the occasional sin and harm nobody else in the doing, so be it. You might die five years younger, but live 15 years happier! Or live five years longer simply because you are happy.

Remember these four simple rules in life:
1. For every action, there is a consequence.
2. If you choose to act, you choose the consequence, be it negative or positive.
3. The choice remains yours and yours alone to make.
4. If you don't choose yourself, then the choice will be made for you by default.

So what choices are you making?

Acceptance, Faith and Gratitude

Being able to accept what you can't change is perhaps the most important quality a person may develop. It works hand in hand with gratitude to guide you through your darkest hours.

But how do you develop acceptance?

By starting small and close to home, and then taking your sphere of acceptance into larger and larger domains.

Being grateful also starts with the very small, being gracious for every breath, every pleasurable experience, every chance to love, to laugh, to live and to learn, however hard the times.

Acceptance, faith and gratitude help you to live with what you cannot change and help you realise that the world sometimes is bigger than you are. Whether your current life situation is the result of random events, or perhaps the Universe dealing you necessary lessons, accepting where you are right now will help ease the struggle.

These are the qualities (along with a Sense of Humour) that will help you deal with the world, when all arguments and positive reasoning come to naught.

SECTION 2

Changing Your Life from Head to Toe

Isn't it ironic? There are so many ways to transform your life, but it is so hard to get one of them right. What makes change difficult is not necessarily the goal itself but the fact that the rest of life keeps intruding on your intention to change. You're concentrating emphatically on controlling your diet. Couldn't your work commitments and family troubles take a break from interrupting your eight-week wonder diet? And could that voice of low self-esteem luring you towards the chocolate bar please quieten down until you've got your waist size under control? Of course not. All of life goes on during any singular period of change. To optimise health, there are so many areas to work on. You have a choice to focus on one specific area of life intently, with a detailed formula to get just one thing right, and hope all else does not drag you down in the doing; or you can look at life in total, and make the simplest changes you can to improve your overall wellbeing.

Small simple steps across a range of health needs, rather than complex single interventions in a specific area of your life.

These two approaches lead to two very different outcomes. You can choose either singular perfection out of balance with the remainder of your life—the perfect body in the broken home, the successful job with a failing heart—or you can choose a balanced approach to life and work, friendship, love and happiness.

Which do you choose? We choose loving life. All of life, in every way …

1

Loving Your Self, Loving Life

From this moment forth, forget all of what has been and how you have seen yourself.

Today is the next moment in loving your Self and loving your Life.

It doesn't matter what traumas you have seen. What weight you are. How many exercise programs you have tried to start and failed to finish. How you've previously felt about yourself, perhaps because of those failures.

History, at this point, means nothing. What we ask you to do is to judge yourself only on what you are going to become. And no, we don't want you to create some outlandish aspiration or fantasy to uplift yourself for the moment. We are not going to set you up for future self-criticism here.

All we want you to consider is simply this: you are going to become better.

Better than what? Better than you are now. That is all.

Can you think that far ahead?

To a moment in which you are better than you are now?

And what does 'better' mean?

Tomorrow it may simply mean a healthier attitude to life. A few well-chosen meals. A walk for exercise. Some sleep preparation. A few more moments of laughter than usual. A pleasure activity, just for you.

Any one of these simple activities might make tomorrow better than today.

So what does that mean about the potential in your life?

It means you have the potential to make your life better. In simple ways, day by day. Grand changes are nice and they may even be necessary. But any small positive change is enough to make life better.

Is there a lot you need to change? If so, then you have the potential for greatness! So much potential to improve. So much potential to celebrate every gain.

You need to take every change as it comes. And love some element of what you are changing and the way it makes you feel. For in loving the change, you are learning to love yourself. And in learning to love yourself, you are learning to love life. Why is this important?

Because if you don't love the potential in your life, if you don't love yourself, you will always be at risk of emotional setback. Negative emotions can set back any one of your health creating goals.

Emotional eating will set your diet back. Learning to love the body you have for what it is becoming, the potential it provides for you to be energetic, vibrant, toned, able to be physically active, is therefore essential.

On the other hand, looking at the body that you have now, before you start to change, and constantly reflecting on its imperfections will eventually drag you down. Why? Because most health enhancing changes come slowly, allowing the evils of a negative body image time to haunt you.

Emotional apathy will set you back. Feeling down because things aren't going right for you now will eventually have you saying, 'Why bother exercising? Why bother trying a relaxation technique? Why bother getting up and enjoying life?'

Why, in fact, should you bother doing anything?

Here's our simple answer. Because life has the potential to turn out for the better. By choosing to get up and do something you enjoy you will be making yourself feel happier. The same goes for exercise, relaxation or any other positive response. Life will be better and therefore you will be happier.

So which do **YOU** choose? To love the potential in your life for betterment? Or to lose your chance at making things better than they are now through continued negative judgement upon the less-than-perfect aspects in your life?

Remember, you can make your life a lot worse in a moment by throwing whatever good you have achieved away, but it usually takes time to bring about concrete positive change. That is why it is so easy to sabotage healthy lifestyle programs. Or is it?

This depends upon you. Do you have an all or nothing attitude towards healthy self-growth? Are you unable to love yourself through the bad as much as the good? And do you throw it all away, the baby with the bath water so to speak, with one mistake?

If so, take the pressure off yourself. Love your mistakes as much as your victories. Allow yourself the small slip-ups. Better still, enjoy them as long as you don't hurt yourself or others permanently in the bargain. For while the overall commitment to the simple health principles in this book will literally add years to your life, both in happiness, health and longevity, no one incident of disobedience, for want of a better term, is going to do irreversible harm.

No one can love their life if they see themselves bound to a torturous and imprisoning path, however health enhancing the supposed benefits. But you can love your life if instead you see yourself as a healthy, happy person exploring and experiencing a few occasions of weakness now and then.

So remember this from the first: 90 per cent is all right.

In fact, if you are only adhering to 10 per cent of the healthy principles in this book, you are more likely to stick to 20 per cent tomorrow, making you even closer to the goals of health and happiness. Perhaps you can adhere to 30 per cent the day or week after. The important concept here is to keep moving, keep taking action.

And love yourself for taking up a little of your personal potential, even if it is not the perfection few, if anyone, will ever achieve anyway. So the lesson is:

Learn to love the potential in your life, rather than the lack.

This said, having given yourself permission to love yourself so simply, there are a few other ways to build on this new-found self love:

- ✦ Nurture yourself every day, by obeying the Pleasure Principle.
- ✦ Be honest and true. To yourself. To others.

- ✦ Constantly seek to understand life, and through understanding, seek self betterment.
- ✦ Find interests in the world that you can be passionate about.
- ✦ Do not compare yourself to others, or to societal images of health or success. You need only please yourself. You need only be content with your own actions.
- ✦ Realise your worth through the intention of actions rather than the outcomes. You cannot control everything in life. So do not scorn yourself for outcomes that were beyond your control.
- ✦ Surround yourself with excellence, with people who support your worth. We have heard it said that the best way to judge a man is by the friends he chooses to keep. Do your friends support your self growth? And remember that what applies to your friends applies tenfold to your intimate partner.
- ✦ Live to your personal principles. If you need to take time out to define your principles, do so, so you know the type of person you wish to love yourself being.
- ✦ Take personal responsibility for the choice of whom you listen to, learn from and follow. Choose role models that will help make you shine.
- ✦ Seek relationships with aspects of life that are greater than your immediate surrounds, and through this, gain a universal perspective on the importance of personal events.

Finally, loving your Self, loving life, has a momentum of its own. That momentum will grow as long as you nurture the emotion. Focus on it. Change your perspectives to foster it, drawing energy away from the destructive emotions—shame, self blame, negative body image, self loathing. Rejoice in each small step on your path towards ultimate self-improvement until focus is no longer necessary and the love of self and life are so deeply entrenched within you, that they are you.

Always remember that you do not need to be 100 per cent perfect to love yourself and your life 100 per cent. You simply need to know that you have the potential to grow one small step at a time.

2

Emotions, Reason, Action

To live is to witness change. There is no way of avoiding it. Change will come, whether you like it or not.

To live well is to direct change; to institute as much control of your life as is necessary, while in turn accepting and even enjoying, where possible, the changes that come, regardless of your efforts.

Your health and happiness are dependent upon directing change. A life without direction is destined for, at best, a slow decline. Health and happiness come with effort, even if it is only the effort to master our emotions to help us achieve a peaceful state of self acceptance, confidence and gratitude.

Most of us, however, want more than this. We would like to move towards a healthier body, better relationships, a successful career, and none of this will happen without choosing to master change, which in turn implies mastering the emotions.

What do we mean here by mastering the emotions?

Not what you might first interpret by this statement. Mastering the emotions does not mean subduing them as if emotions were not important. On the contrary, emotions are the most important quality in our lives.

We act only from our emotions. We are always seeking positive emotions. Emotions are the reward for achieving what we want in life.

It doesn't matter if you are getting a promotion, buying a car, greedily enjoying the figure in your bank account or your first kiss, it is the internalised result of these events that drives you towards enjoying them; happiness, joy, contentment, love, indulgence.

Negative emotions also play an essential part in our lives. They may also drive us towards acting for positive outcomes. All negative emotions have a purpose when consistent with the events that cause them. Anger and aggression may save your life when threatened, sadness and depression slow you down in order to assess a situation and understand the loss of what you value and contemplate your response.

However, emotions are primitive responses designed around a simpler world. Physical aggression was once appropriate in many situations; anger backed with verbal and physical strength was essential to ensuring you remained healthy, and through surviving, happy. But times have changed. The world is now different.

It has literally become a far more 'reasonable' place, where rational responses are often required to address situations and, as a result, emotions need to be placed in appropriate context. The world of commerce and finance, business in any form, law and education, even such comparatively 'primitive' areas as agriculture and mining, rely upon objective reasoning, calculation and rule of law if a person is to interact successfully within these spheres. Even personal health has become dominated by a medical world of measures and tests.

This overwhelming turn towards science and reason in the world of work and even our personal lives has had wholesale implications for the attunement of our emotions throughout our lives, and our ability to keep them in context with what we are doing. What does this have to do with our simple health and happiness book? Everything! What we are trying to highlight is the increased complexity and even alienation many of us battle with when putting our emotions and reasoning in context and how this comes back to haunt even our simplest of decisions.

Without maturely addressing our emotions and reason concerning any area in which we want to change our lives, we risk sabotaging every outcome we attempt to influence.

We need to understand and work with our emotions if we are to be satisfied with life, simply because satisfaction with life is ultimately experienced through the emotions.

However, emotions only provide us with the impulse to change events; they do not necessarily guide us towards sensible responses. This is therefore why we need reason.

How does this impact upon your life, and how in turn can you make simple practical changes to direct you towards health and happiness with every emotion you experience?

The answer lies in developing skills to take command of the chain of events between an experience and an emotionally aware response, rather than allowing your reaction to be a reflexive, habitual response.

Consider the following example. Your partner gets angry at you for a simple mistake. How you perceive their anger will depend upon your system of personal beliefs, as learnt from your individual interpretation of previous experience and/ or other teachings. This perception will filter through your own personal temperament towards a reaction. But here is the critical moment.

Are you going to re-act or act? Are you going to reflexively respond, or rather are you going to act with reasonable awareness?

You might reflexively argue back about the many mistakes your partner has made, escalating the tension and decide that your partner doesn't care enough about you. You might then consider whether or not this is actually due to your figure, emotionally eat and decide you could not be bothered with exercising today. Light up a cigarette instead. Storm out and go for a drink. One drink turns to nine. A fight with a stranger at the bar. Drink drive home ...

One simple argument. And a small ripple of emotion turns into an eventual tidal wave affecting your whole life. You might think this is an extreme example. It is (although many people do follow the whole path or some similar chain of events). But how far do you go through a chain of reflexive events before a moment of contemplative reasoning steps in to identify that this whole series of emotionally driven behaviours is disproportionate to what has started the initial emotion in the first place?

Such a series of reflexive actions only needs a moment of reasonable contemplation to stop its momentum. A moment in which you take a deep breath, realise that the anger you are feeling is simply and singularly related to a degree of annoyance at your partner's lack of understanding over your mistake. A concern that, in an appropriate moment, you can address (be it now or later) but not one that calls for an emotional attack of your own, followed by emotionally driven feeding, smoking and drinking behaviours and concluding in an abandonment of anything positive in your life (your exercise program, healthy eating plan and expensive plates—how often are you actually arguing about the crockery you break?)

So how do you change the way you address your life, so that you can guide all change by taking command over your re-actions, making them instead contemplative, reasonable actions?

The first step is to understand what drives your emotions in the first place. And that is the interrelationship between your **temperament** and your **perception** in any particular circumstance.

Let us first look at your temperament. Are you generally aggressive, balanced depending on circumstances or, at the other extreme, subdued? Either extreme may present a problem in the wrong circumstance. Meaning, if you have only one response to a crisis, to get angry or to back down, sooner or later you will find yourself in a situation in which your response is inappropriate. The reality is, there will be times when anger is appropriate and times when backing down and negotiating is appropriate.

Can you work on your temperament to develop a mature level of flexibility? Yes, although it is beyond the scope of this particular book to discuss in great detail.

A first step if you are of an angry or even excessively assertive temperament, is to work on relaxation techniques and acceptance, then enrol yourself into Anger Management 101. It really is worth it, because an angry or overly assertive temperament is destructive to most aspects of your life.

If you are of the subdued temperament, look at working on self-esteem, optimism and most importantly, enrol yourself in Assertiveness Training 102 as soon as possible. Simply because if you cannot assert yourself, then the chances of changing anything in your life are minimal.

The second influence on your emotions is how you perceive an event. What do you believe about it?

Do you automatically believe what your partner is saying in an angered moment, regardless of the truth in it, or, on reflection, do you perceive the situation differently?

This choice is yours depending on what you wish to perceive.
So what do you do if you want to perceive a subject or event differently?

Change what you believe about it.

Is your partner right, that you are 'good for nothing' because you made a mistake? We've seen above the negative behaviours that can escalate when we re-act to such a comment.

But stop for a moment. Stop before you take on such a negative reaction and ask the most important question of all. Is your partner actually right?

Only if you choose to believe him or her. You could simply believe instead that your partner is angry. And know that in moments of anger, any number of unjustified statements may be made, even by someone who loves you. You made one mistake, amongst many otherwise perfect performances for the day. Your partner will get over it. They might just have had a bad day themselves. Give them a little space and wait until the emotions or situation have been somewhat diffused. Prepare that healthy dinner, then go back and suggest you exercise together. Talk about the issues after the stress response has been burnt out.

Do you see how a different belief regarding your partner's anger has changed your perception of the event, and hence your response. Why? Because …

Your beliefs can change your perception of reality, and your subsequent actions, based on those beliefs, can change reality itself. So choose your beliefs carefully. Don't let them choose you.

Choose to interpret situations differently. Choose only to believe what others say (whether in spoken or written form, personal words or those written in a text book) if you want to, or have to because it is undeniable fact. Remember that especially when it comes to relationships, most of what is said is interpretation and not fact, even when people confidently assert something as such. If you don't believe the source of information, look for another source or interpretation.

The skill of being able to live in the moment directly applies here also. Try to maintain perspective in such situations. If it helps you may imagine yourself rising above your body, moving a little further on in time and jumping back down to a time when the heat of the moment is over, emotions are more settled and laughter may even be on its way. If this works for you, teach your partner and life will be better one thousandfold with a minimum of effort.

And what should you do with the emotions that arise?

First, identify the emotions and assess them for consistency.

These are Lessons One and Two in the science of Emotional Intelligence.

Do you actually know what emotion you are feeling at any given time? Do you recognise your emotions as they are building or only when they explode forth in violent rage, abusive anger or overwhelming anxiety? Do you skip dissatisfaction, and even sadness, and only realise your pain once in the depths of depression?

Here is an exercise, particularly pertinent if the above paragraph applies to you. Whenever you feel an emotion rising in intensity, stop and name it. Do nothing else. Simply identify what you are feeling. It is important to be as specific as possible.

Say it. I feel angry. I feel sad. I feel disappointed. Rejected. Jealous. Shamed. Blamed. Guilty. In danger.

Look at this list of emotions. Every one of these emotions might simply have been identified as a reason to feel angry. But every one of them calls for its own appropriate response.

Have you ever met a person who gets angry at everything? There is usually a simple reason why. They have very few other emotional responses in life as they misidentify almost all negative emotions as anger. If they feel disappointed, they get angry; if they feel sad, they get angry; if they feel jealous, they get angry. They only get angry. Therefore they never can address disappointment, sadness or jealousy, and hence have even more reason to get angry! But if they begin to identify these emotions for what they actually are, all of a sudden a whole new world of appropriate expression is available to them. They can then use disappointment as motivation, or sadness as a period to reflect on values and redirect their life, for example. Through identifying a whole range of appropriate emotions, with, in turn, an equally appropriate set of mature responses they can begin to experience less anger.

The next consideration is whether or not the emotion is consistent with what has elicited it. It may not be. Maybe the emotion has rolled on from a previous circumstance. Or perhaps you are running an internal program built up from a past experience that only barely resembles this present moment. We all contain such unconscious programs that guide many of our reflexive responses (again, beyond the scope of this particular book to discuss).

What to do with the inconsistency?

Stop. Identify it.

AND DON'T REACT TO IT!

Take a deep breath. Take a few deep breaths. Walk away for a moment if you are angry and about to act on your anger. Or stand firm if you are about to flee. Stop your hand reaching reflexively for the emotionally driven chocolate biscuit, cigarette or vodka bottle.

This is the moment for contemplative reasoning. This is the time to think life through. This is the moment of choice. You have at least two options; to react with your emotions or to act through reason. In fact, with the second choice there are likely to be many options. While acting on our emotions sends us down only one path, reason gives us a multitude. That is why reasoning gives you freedom.

This can only be said of true reasoning, however, preceded by both an act of awareness of our emotions and an awareness of the consequences of our actions.

And the ultimate consequences of our actions are the emotions that result. Therefore in order to achieve the greatest happiness as derived from the greatest life outcomes we need to choose the most positive action that we can reasonably make, given any situation in our lives.

Do you follow a whole sea of reactive actions set loose upon a broken dam of emotions? Or do you isolate the true reason for the emotion, respond to the situation with reasonable action that in turn generates the most positive consequence, and hence most positive change, and finally the greatest ocean of positive emotions possible?

It is important that we learn to identify and understand our emotions and reason if we want to be happy. Rationality without resort to happiness is pointless, at least as far as fulfilling one's own life is concerned, while living by our emotions will only lead to volatile and unstable living. To live successfully we therefore need to respect both emotion and reason. So here is a practical path to balancing emotion, reason, action and change. Whenever you feel a growth in negative emotion, or, more directly, are confronted by a stressful challenge, short of physical attack:

STOP!

Take however many **DEEP BREATHS** are required to **CALM THE MIND**. Walk away if you have to. Apologise for the need to be absent if necessary. Return only when calmed.

DO NOT REACT BEFORE YOU FEEL IN COMMAND OF YOUR EMOTIONS!

IDENTIFY THE EMOTION with an exact title (broaden your vocabulary of emotions as much as possible).

IDENTIFY WHY YOU FEEL THE EMOTION, and the **CONSISTENCY OF THE EMOTION**.

CONSIDER as many reasoned **RESPONSES** as possible. **DISCUSS** the issue if necessary.

ACT WITH AWARENESS OF OUTCOMES you wish to achieve that lead to the happiest, healthiest, most life satisfying consequences.

And additionally, at a later point, work on the **TEMPERAMENT** and **BELIEF STRUCTURE** that led you to the initial emotion in the first place.

This is contemplative reasoning in touch with your emotions. At first it will be a slightly punctuated mode of action but eventually it will become a subconscious process if you use it often enough. Before you reflexively heighten your emotion in response to an argument with a partner or cower away from a necessary discussion with a "superior".

Before you reach for the cigarette packet or duck into the corner store for the serve of fried chips.

Think Perception-Emotion-Reason-Action-Consequence and choose to turn the emotions that arise into happiness and health that abounds!

3

Building Better Relationships

It is time to answer the following question: What, amongst the whole of your life, other than your own personal wellbeing, is most important to you?

Second question: Who, other than yourself, is most important to you?

Did you come up with the same answer?

If not, should you have?

The reality is, as a human you are fundamentally a social being. Short of the rare psychopath or two, you are basically built to relate. Relationships with others are a primary part of not only your quest for happiness, but your ability to be healthy as well. For most of us, the greatest desire in life is to have a fulfilling relationship with a loving partner, to watch our children grow and to receive the acknowledgement and acceptance of our parents, whether or not they agree with our choice of lifestyle.

Countless studies, as recounted for example in Dr Dean Ornish's work *Love and Survival—The Scientific Basis for the Healing Power of Intimacy*, attest to the fact that the state of our relationships play a large part in not only whether we are happy in life, but whether or not we will suffer illness as well. Not just the relationships we have with immediate family either, but also our relationships with our friends, support groups, community in general and even our pets. In fact, one study showed dogs help lower blood pressure more than good friends!

But you know that, don't you? You don't need a study to prove this. You're always feeling better with your family and partner supporting you and your dog at your feet.

So you must be giving your family relationships the highest priority in your life other than yourself, mustn't you? Or are you?

For so many, this simply is not the case. Why? Perhaps it is the pressure of our modern society. The need to succeed. To own. To invest. But what are we doing all this for? Does success, ownership, financial security or any other activity precede the importance of your relationships? Are they more important than your relationship with your partner, your children, your parents?

Be honest, what would you want more, an intimate relationship with your partner or a better career, greater financial security, a bigger house or faster car?

What about your relationship with your children?

Who among you would consciously choose to sacrifice the quality of your relationship with your children, even if you unconsciously do so time and time again, as many of us do?

If the career, the financial security, the bigger house or faster car comes first, chances are, you are in the wrong relationship! And if you are willing to sacrifice your children, well ... we'll leave that to your own interpretation.

So ask yourself honestly, do you give your partner and family the highest priority in your life?

Not would you ... but do you already? Now! Every day. In the small decisions that you make? Between extra overtime to pay off a bigger house versus time with the kids? Do you think they prefer the bigger house or time with you more? Between playing golf on weekends or spending valuable time patching up your relationship with your partner after a hard week?

Do you consciously decide to value your relationships first?

Your family first?

And not what the family owns, where the family goes, what the family does, but how the family relates to each other.

Relationships matter. And not just with family either. Relationships matter, be they friendships, community or even the workplace. In fact the modern age has raised the work relationship to a level where the time we spend with work mates may be greater than that with our intimate partners!

So here is a special life quest.

Put relationships first. Strive for quality relationships in your life. Don't take them for granted. Honour them.

How can you do this? By making a conscious decision to reflect on how you can improve on the quality of your relationships on a daily basis. Focusing on every relationship to begin with might be hard, so here is a suggestion. Every day, before starting your day's activities, focus on two or three relationships and consider for a brief moment how you could most improve each of these relationships. We suggest first focusing on:

1. Your relationship with your partner
2. Your relationship with your children
3. Your relationship with your parents
4. The next 2–3 people who you will spend the most time with on that day, or at least the most vital moments with, even if not paralleled by the amount of time spent
5. Alternatively, consider a person who you feel you have not been as close to of late as you would like

Now, before you start to worry that you are about to sacrifice your life to others in focusing on your relationships in such a way, think again. Relationships are about how you relate to others, not how you surrender your life to them. This quest is to improve how you relate to others. Therefore, while increasing the quality time you dedicate to a relationship may be one action, there are a multitude of other emotionally intelligent ways to improve your dealings with others, ranging from improving communication and developing empathy, to giving others space, or even ending a dysfunctional relationship.

This again comes down to developing the skill set known as Emotional Intelligence. What follows are some of the emotional intelligence skills you could try to develop in response to the relationships you are focusing on daily.

Tick which are most appropriate for you to develop:

☐ **Recognising Others' Emotions:** How well do you read what other people feel? Are you observant of others' emotions? Or do you interact with people as a one person wrecking ball, failing to read what people feel? If so, it's time to begin to watch the way those around you express their emotions. Are they reserved, bottling everything up, or do they need to be watched in case they explode into a sea of emotion?

☐ **Managing Others' Emotions:** Once you have identified others' emotions, are you able to react with empathy and compassion towards their sadness? Are you able to manage their behaviour before they explode? The more you learn to manage others' emotions, the more you will be able to successfully negotiate the minefield of consequences that such emotions can create.

☐ **Communication Skills:** Do you feel your relationships are developed upon clear communication lines? Do others hear not only what you are saying, but what you are actually meaning? Do you need to be more direct in what you say, or more subtle? Do you listen well AND comprehend the hidden meaning in tone and pitch, as well as the largely unspoken word conveyed in non-verbal communications (body language)? If you are constantly having battles with people over issues you predominantly agree on (strange how this happens, isn't it?), look at how you are communicating your message (both verbally and non-verbally), for you are probably making even bigger mistakes when your ideas are actually in conflict.

☐ **Clearly Define and Identify Your Own and Others' Boundaries:** Do you establish and communicate clear boundaries in your relationships? Are people aware of the ways you wish them to interact with you? Do you say 'No' and get heard? Or do you fail to assert your personal needs? Do you respect the ways people want to interact with you and the ways they don't? Do you hear them say 'No' to you? Or do you lack a respect for others' boundaries? Are you willing to say 'Yes' to helping other people who are in (appropriate) need or are you too selfish? Are you willing to hear the 'Yes' of others' willingness to help you, or are you too proud?

If you fail in any of these areas, it is time to improve how you relate to others and hence the quality of your relationships by learning to establish clear boundaries.

☐ **Understand Rules:** This overlaps with defining your boundaries. But rules are the small print. Understanding the personal idiosyncrasies of relationships as they develop is knowing the rules. This takes constant communication with others, asking such questions as necessary to define each person's personal likes and dislikes.

☐ **Show Interest:** Now this is simple. Do you actually show interest in others? Do you make their life, their opinion, their existence feel important? We all want to feel important. It helps our self-esteem. And when you make others feel important, they will return the favour ... with interest. So show interest!

☐ **Know Your Appropriate Relationship Management Styles:** Do you attempt to manage everyone with the same style?
Are you a managing director at work, on the sports field, at home, at the bar, in the bedroom? And should you be?
Of course not. Developing an awareness of appropriate management styles in different life situations is important, particularly in transitioning between work and how we relate to our partners and children.

☐ **Learn to Understand Others' Perspectives:** Try to understand how it would be in another's shoes. How they think, how they feel, what they actually want. This will make you far more effective in not only reading what is being communicated, but what is wanted by another person. If you do not think you can do this, or want to know if you are doing it well, simply ask others what they are thinking, feeling, wanting.

☐ **Develop Win-Win Conflict Resolution Strategies:** Seek to identify how everyone can best be served by an outcome, rather than simply seeking selfishly for yourself in any circumstance.

Negotiate bargains for all, that work to foster continued community partnerships. Win-win solutions are not always possible in situations of direct competition, but they should be worked towards.

☐ **Understand Group Dynamics:** Learn how to be diplomatic and get the most out of group situations. Realise the loudest person is not always the one who should get the most attention. Knowing how to extract the most from any group is a vital talent to develop.

☐ **Constantly Monitor Your Relationship States:** Become vigilant in assessing the state of your relationships. Become aware of where they are heading. And when there are problems, learn to identify what they are as soon as possible so they may be addressed. This also includes realising when relationships should end, or at least be redefined. Some relationships are not healthy for us, at least as they stand at present.

☐ **Learn to Forgive (which does not necessarily mean forgetting):** Forgiveness is the ultimate step towards the resolution of negative emotion. While negative emotions remain hidden within, they may continue to haunt our physical, emotional and even rational sides of our Mindbody. Forgiveness does not imply opening ourselves up to further abuse. It is first and foremost a personal closure and does not need to involve another party, particularly where it is safer to stay away from the potential for further hurt.

☐ **And Ask For Forgiveness:** This, too, is a search for personal closure. The least you can do is ask and understand your own regret. But asking for forgiveness should also include a commitment to improve, so that you do not need to be forgiven again in the future. Otherwise, it is a half-hearted act at best, and at worst, an act of deception.

Which will you choose to work on tomorrow?

4

Living with Passion

The modern world can so easily overwhelm us. Successful job or not, we can be run from pillar to post serving other's commands in return for a pay cheque. It might be idealistic to believe we can all be working in a job that matches our life's desires, but this is often not the case. Yet, at the end of the day or week there is something we can do about this.

We can find some time to dedicate to fulfilling our own personal passion.

Perhaps on a weeknight, perhaps during our time off, but sometime during the week, at least once a week and for a meaningful period of time, you should work upon an act of **self-creation**. An act that makes you feel whole and fulfilled. A task that fills you with pride, leaving you able to say, I have done something that makes me experience what it personally feels like to be completely alive!

Don't mistake this with the list of tasks we have committed you to in the name of the Pleasure Principle. No, we are looking for a unique, or set of unique, life desires, that form a subgroup of pleasure activities that you enjoy. Activities that you more than enjoy, activities that you live for. Activities that you are passionate about. So you not only now have a Pleasure Principle, you also have a **Passion Principle**.

> *I am a Passionate Being.*
> *I choose to fulfil my passions as best as I can.*
> *I therefore dedicate myself to find,*
> *as often as possible,*
> *a meaningful period of time*
> *for my Passions …*

Remember, this is **YOUR** time. Yes, your partner, your children may be your passion, and we have ensured accounting for them in the previous chapter. But this is not what we mean here. This is **YOUR** time, for **YOUR** passions. Because ...

You deserve to change the world, too!

Do you know what your passion is?
Is it creating beautiful pieces of art, sculpture, pottery?
Is it collecting?
Have you heightened the love of a sport to a passion?
Is travelling a passion for you?
Writing?
Learning about history, space travel or quantum science?
Rebuilding a car?
Creating a beautiful garden?
In other words, what do you value doing AND being good at?

Throughout your life it is in the best interests of your health if you continue to be passionate about and **ACT** on one or more of your personal passions at any one time.

So what are you working on now?

If you have paused here and not come up with an answer, it is time to find one.

NOW! AND ACT ON IT NOW!

So we have looked at pleasure and we have looked at passion, but there is one more step beyond to work towards.

Turning Your Passion into Your Employment

This is what we should all strive for in life. To be paid to do something we are passionate about, or at the very least, something we enjoy. This is what we should consider as often as possible, in order to achieve greatest life satisfaction. How can life not be fulfilling, when time at work is nothing more, but also nothing less, than play? Imagine coming home thinking that even if you weren't paid to do what you are doing, you'd still love to do it!

Therein is perhaps one of the greatest challenges in life.

But how to do it? Here are two simple approaches that certainly overlap.

The first is to have faith. Be clear with your intentions and actions, create new paths, keep your eyes open, take some risks and welcome the chance to follow your passions head on. Make the leap of faith with one almighty jump!

The second option is a more gradual and rational approach. Consider how in small ways you can make the transition. Perhaps one day a week, or even in your spare time. Little by little. But don't hold back all the same. Whenever you are dedicating yourself to the task, live it with passion. And all of a sudden, as people realise the intensity of your application, passion will drive you on to greater things. And suddenly the small half chance will be the big opportunity, for people love working with those who are passionate.

Meanwhile, here's a little trick to get you through the less than passionate parts of your workday and week. Perhaps, at this moment, you work nine to five, five days a week plus overtime. In fact, the longer this time frame is in your life, the more important you find a solution. And the trick is to invest yourself in what you are doing now. Live it as if it is your passion. You have to be at work anyway, so why not enjoy it?

Find ways to be passionate about the non-passionate parts of your life. Do whatever you can to make the less than interesting parts of life more interesting, with the only proviso being that you do not lose competence in whatever actually needs to be done.

On the other hand, don't complain about what you are doing, unless you are prepared to stop doing it. Otherwise, you are simply reinforcing the pain of not being passionate about your role. Furthermore, by concentrating on the lack in your life, you will surely continue to live it.

So the key to life is to make it as passionate as possible, even if you have to initially fake it to make it.

And if you think the latter suggestion is an artificial way of living your life to make it pleasurable, well it is. But only as long as it takes to get you to a place of living with genuine passion.

Which is far less damaging an approach than the other artificial ways of making you happy in life. What are they? Alcohol, recreational drugs, smoking, emotional eating and other behavioural excesses. So which do you choose?

5

Towards Stress-less Living

Stress. You know what it is! It's the consequence of living in our fast paced, don't stop, must be successful society. The feelings experienced when the pressures of life overwhelm and threaten to come caving in.

And you know what it does to you as well, we're sure. Increases your risk of heart disease, ulcers, high blood pressure and having a stroke ... need we go on? Hopefully that won't be the case for you in five, ten or twenty years' time.

Right now it is simply making you unhappy!

And that is good enough reason to take action and reduce the stress, or at least the effects of stress, upon your life.

So, what causes stress?
Any threat to the value in your life. That threat could be physical, emotional, financial, or social. The result is the same. You feel stressed.

What is your response to stress? Your heart rate increases, your muscles tighten, your stomach temporarily stops digesting food, while your immune system takes a temporary back seat.

Why? You're getting ready to run, fight or hide. The case is the same whether the situation of stress is a person trying to assault you, a problem with your finances, or you're becoming nervous about an interview.

Now running, fighting or hiding may be an effective way of dealing with an aggressor, but not necessarily your finances or an interview. And so to the problem of the primitive human stress response.

Problem Number 1: Your body's stress response is designed to deal with physical danger. Many modern stressors, however, are not of a physical nature. They are instead related to emotional, financial or moral dilemmas.

Problem Number 2: Your body's stress response is designed to be enacted only for short periods of time as required for running or fighting (seconds or minutes). Modern stressors, of a non-physical nature, however, may take hours, days or even months to resolve.

Outcome: Rather than experiencing short, sharp and manageable increases in heart rate, respiratory rate, blood pressure and so forth, prolonged stress perpetuates health issues due to the continued effects of the ongoing stress response. Leading to increased risk of heart disease, high blood pressure, infection and other immune system dysfunctions and digestive problems such as ulcers, to name only a few.

Of course that is not to forget the even more obvious effects on your general sense of wellbeing and, taken to the point of dis-ease, clinical anxiety and depression with the subsequent impact on self-esteem, motivation, emotional eating patterns and so forth.

High stress living is not good for your health! So what is stressing you?

This is a personal question. For what stresses you is different to what stresses us. It's individual.

Why? Because the amount of stress we feel is dependent upon what we value, how we perceive the world and our place in it, and what skills, resources and time we have to change the outcomes in our life.

The first question is: **Do You Know What is Stressing You?**

This is a very simple question. Yes, you might know, for example, that there is something about your relationship with your partner that is annoying you, but what exactly is it? How clearly can you define the problem? This is important because you can't act to eliminate the stress if you only vaguely know what is upsetting you. But after identifying the problem you can work on solutions, and solutions are the only way you are going to ultimately stop your stress.

Strangely enough, we often find that what is stressing us is simply an annoyance, rather than a big issue. This is particularly the case when multiple small irritations build throughout the day. Each irritation alone, identified, and dealt with or accepted for what it is, becomes of little significance. But if each independent annoyance is allowed to breed on the previous annoyance—growing into irritation, frustration, anger—it will culminate ultimately in a stress explosion. This is why your proverbial cat gets a kick at the end of the day, even if you love him in the morning. He is the outlet of your terrible day of small annoyances.

So the key is to identify what is stressing you.

And put a value on it. For if you identify what you are stressing over as of little value to you, why bother stressing over it? As the title of a successful self-help book so aptly puts it, 'Don't Sweat the Small Stuff'. And most of it is small stuff!

Therefore, if what stresses you is of little value, take a deep breath, and shift the problem from your focus.

Your next step after evaluating your stress is to decide whether you should be stressing over a problem even if what is at stake is of value to you. Maybe what you are stressing over isn't an issue. How could this be the case?

Well, take a common example. Here's a worry for you. You made a mistake at work today and your mind is racing ... *'I'm going to lose my job, the customers are going to tell the boss what I said, the boss will relay it up the management chain ... I'm a goner! ... then I won't be able to pay the bills ... and what will my partner think ...?'*

But is any of this actually going to happen? Is it predestined reality or your perceptions gone wild? Is what you are thinking based on fact or the mind chatter from a host of voices inside your head seeking out every worst case scenario they can find? Did the customer actually hear what you said? Did they even care? Even if they did, could they be bothered telling the boss? Will the boss care? Will it matter since you have brought in ten other clients?

There are a lot of possible steps that must occur if your concern is to come true. But all you are considering is the worst case scenario.

Do you know it is estimated that only 10 per cent of what you worry about relates to events or circumstances that will actually happen?

Wouldn't it be nice to only worry about the 10 per cent that does happen rather than the 90 per cent that doesn't? That would be a start, wouldn't it?

And this start will only happen if you learn to differentiate between perceptions built upon past experience or erroneous learning, and realistic interpretations based on present fact.

Do you do this? Think about it for a moment. Choose the area in life you stress over most to answer the question. The area of your life you are least secure about. What effect do your insecurities have on your perceptions of the events to come?

And how do you stop this from becoming the case? The answer is, gather in the information. Check it out. Make decisions upon the facts. And if you can't be objective yourself, ask for an independent opinion from a person who will give an unbiased answer.

Meanwhile, go back to those Emotional Intelligence skills and work on clarifying your perceptions in the areas in which they are most clouded (which will most likely correlate with the areas in your life in which you are most stressed).

So, what about the 10 per cent of life worth stressing over?

What can you do about these situations?

Simple: **Find Solutions.**

That is how you eliminate stress. You overcome the challenge.

In fact let us overcome the word 'stress'. You're now 'challenged' instead!

And how do you practically overcome a challenge?

Through applying the following resources:

Finances, Time and Skills. These are the three primary inputs required to overcome any challenge.

Unfortunately, much of the modern world involves money. Money buys 'things', money buys skills, money accesses more money.

So you really need to get your money in order. As simple as that. Go see an accountant or financial advisor and balance the budget. However much you want to argue that it is not what makes the world go round, if you abuse your finances, it is what will make the world come to your door ... angry, and willing to take your house, your car and your sanity.

Overcome your belief that money is an evil if you have it. It is not. Nor is it a god worth worshipping and losing your life to. It is simply a value system.

See it for what it is. Paper and metal that simply put a value on what you want. It purchases the time you value, the skills you value and the things you value. Money is rarely the real problem in anyone's life, even if you stress over it. The real problem is understanding what you value most, and in turn where you choose to apply what money you have. If you blame money for your stress, you are simply denying personal responsibility for lacking a true understanding of what you value most.

If you work too much because you need the money so you can buy (or, worse, pay off) the 'things' you want in life, the problem is not the money, not the work, but the inconsistency between what you value and how you choose to act in life. Wanting too many 'things' will cost you time at work. You're trading time for 'things', money is just the go-between.

But what else are you losing? The answer is, whatever else you value that you could be doing with the time you spend at work earning the money.

Number one reason for marriage failure at present is? Overwork.

If you contest this answer and instead wish to say 'money', well it's basically much the same answer for most people.

What are you working for? Simple answer, more money. But more money for what? Your house, holiday, family car or luxury items (including a bigger house, longer holiday, faster second family car).

But are the 'things' you are buying with the extra time at work worth the relationship you are losing by not having the time to commit to it?

Even if the 'thing' in question is the family house, is the extra work required worth the risk of losing your relationship?

Not if you value your relationship more than your house (or, in most present-day instances, a bigger, more luxurious family house).

The reality is, overwork and a quest for more money aren't the fundamental problems at the heart of many questions over stress, even if they are the practical considerations that need to be acted on. It is the inability of people to directly draw parallels between what they value most, and the choices they make in life.

And that is fundamentally a question of understanding Life Balance, as much as it is a question of finances.

So the question of money, work and financing comes down to this: If you want to have more money, you will need to earn it. But are the sacrifices you need to make to earn (or save) the extra money worth the loss or risk of devaluing all other aspects of your life necessary to attain that money?

For it is the loss or risk of loss that is going to lead to the stress you feel on a daily basis.

What about the question of time? How does this relate to stress?

That's obvious, isn't it? The second greatest stress in life after overwork/money is time management. Many of us are poor at it. Do you have a Time Management System? Do you know how to **prioritise** your time, so that the necessary is achieved by its deadline date? That's Time Stress Number One, missing deadline dates on essential tasks.

Time Stress Number Two precedes this and is the stress of **meeting** deadline dates (even when you've made them yourself!)

So, how do you avoid both Time Stresses?

Put simply, by choosing to do Important tasks long before they become Deadline tasks (or Urgent tasks). This is healthy time management that prevents stress. It also means delegating Unimportant tasks (e.g. watching television) to either low priority or no priority. In other words, doing these tasks only when all else is done or not doing them at all. Again, like money, the question of time comes back to knowing what you value. Time should be dedicated to what you value most, or need to value because of the way society works (paying your bills, meeting work deadlines).

That is all we wish to say on time management, not because it is of low importance, but that it requires a more thorough examination than we can provide in a simple book. So we will simply say, if you do not use a time management system and find yourself under regular time pressure, your first task after reading this book is to investigate the subject of time management. A good place to start is by reading works by Stephen Covey, from which the brief discussion on Urgent/Important/Not Urgent/Not Important tasks and Time Management is drawn.

Time management is essential not only to stressing less, but also to good health. Put simply, without it you will fail to find the time necessary to commit to exercise, relaxation and healthy meal preparation.

Lastly, to overcome what is stressing you, you will need to develop **appropriate life skills**. Often, it does not matter exactly what is stressing you. But unless you find the particular skills to overcome your problem, it will continue to stress you! It gets no simpler than that.

It does not matter if it is learning a physical task such as erecting a fence, an intellectual task such as brushing up on the latest tax regulations, or an Emotional Intelligence skill such as anger management, impulse control or asserting your personal boundaries; each example represents an essential skill that may need to be developed in order to overcome what is stressing you.

So, once you have identified the stressor, you need to also identify the skills needed to overcome what is stressing you. And commit to learning them. Or delegate them! (if possible)

Now, there is a solution. Delegate! The modern world is extremely complex, and we delegate many of our potential stresses before they even stress us, by paying someone skilled. Rather than stress over repairing the car, we hire a mechanic. Instead of learning medicine or law, we see a doctor or lawyer. Instead of stressing over the cleaning, we hire a cleaner.

The question is, to what extent are you prepared to delegate life chores to others and can you afford to?

Again, this is a question of how much you value avoiding the stress, and how much you are willing to compensate for this by paying someone else to do the task for you. Someone who is not only less stressed doing the task than you, they actually love it! Have you noticed there is always someone who loves doing something you hate to do? The universe is in amazing balance; it creates people obsessed about all sorts of things that need doing!

Don't mock them for it. Fulfil their passion through delegation and their need for employment by paying them to do their passion. Indeed, this is the very wish you want for yourself!

So all three practical resources—finances, time and skills—as well as your perceptions of stress and whether or not you should actually take a stressful circumstance on in the first place, comes back to what you value.

So what is stress?
A threat to that which you value as an individual.
And how do you overcome stress?
By learning to deal effectively with the challenge.

But what if you cannot deal effectively with the challenge now (and have no means of delegating the situation)? You have a fallback position. We call it 'Effects Based Stress Management'. This is what the majority of most stress management approaches are about. The answer, in simple terms, is to put a bandaid on your body and mind, to burn off the effects of stress, even if you are unable to currently address the causes. And in the short-term, as well as for dealing with the mass of minor stressful irritations before they build to major frustrations, Effects Based Stress Management techniques work wonders. What are they?

Simple. You have already been introduced to them throughout this book.

Exercise.

Relaxation.

Choosing to enjoy yourself instead of worry. In other words, the Pleasure Principle and the Passion Principle.

Eating well and keeping yourself healthy enough to take up the challenge.

Maintaining a healthy mind through acceptance, gratitude, optimism and other Emotional Intelligence skills.

Using Simple Healthy Living Principles to burst through stress.

But remember, these are stress management techniques that deal only with the effects of stress. They will not prevent its insidious claws from pulling you back time and time again unless you address the root causes, whatever they personally may be.

For ultimately, you need to take action. Only through action will your life change in the long-term.

Start by making a daily list of the essential tasks you need to do to address the causes of your stress, the challenges that you face. Pay your bills. Do your accounts. Manage your time. Delegate a task to someone. Make a few phone calls that matter. Develop a skill. Take time out to return quality to a relationship. Do something! Pursue as many actions as you can each day to take up the challenge of what is stressing you, so that every day there is less and less residual stresses to worry over.

So we finish this chapter with a Stress Busting Suggestion. Every day, at some point before going to work (the first few minutes after you wake, as you have a shave or shower), make a mental note of at least five actions you are going to undertake to make your life less stressful. Ensure at least three of these actions address the cause of your present stresses and not just the symptoms (i.e. don't just include five effects-based techniques), and include at least one that addresses your greatest present stress.

And during the day ensure you action this list.

If you simply do this every day we can guarantee that your life will begin to change towards a less stressed, more happy and healthy state of Being.

6

To Laugh, To Sing, To Dance, To Make Love

Laugh, and the world laughs with you. In joyous song, with vibrant delight. Could there be a healthier, easier exercise for the complete Being—body, mind and soul—than laughter?

Here is a list of some of the benefits of *laughter...*

- Laughter is the ultimate stress buster, at least as far as effects based stress management goes.
- The longer you laugh, the closer laughter comes to cardiovascular exercise. Laughter clears the stale air from the deeper parts of your lungs.
- Laughter is an instant of happiness, no matter how intense the surrounding pain.
- Laughter relieves pain, working as a natural anaesthetic.
- Laughter is infectious, a magical aid to socialising and making new friends.
- Laughter fights infections, boosting the immune system.
- Laughter increases creativity.
- Laughter battles against mood disorders, anxiety and depression.
- Laughter enhances education, performance and teamwork.

It's a magical drug, a stimulant for happiness, improves work productivity and enlightens the soul. It feels good, is good for you, and costs nothing.

So why aren't you doing more of it?

Take a look at your children. Does it come as any surprise that laughter is only natural to them? Why do they laugh as much as they do and you laugh as much as you don't?

Is it because children have much more fun in childhood than adults do during adultery ... let us rephrase that ... adulthood? Is there anything inherent about being a child that makes you laugh more?

Perhaps. What, then, could this be?

Here's our opinion. It's permission. Permission to laugh. Children are not self-conscious about laughing and what they laugh about. They don't stop to ask themselves constantly, should I be laughing? But adults, on the other hand, look around to see who is watching, assess the quality of the joke to see if it meets our standards, review our environment and so forth, before giving ourselves permission to laugh. And after doing all this, few things are left to laugh about.

So do you give yourself permission to laugh?

Yes or no? With little restraint?

Note, we said little restraint. Yes, there are times that laughing may not be appropriate. It should not be used to dominate, ridicule, exclude or offend.

So what subjects shouldn't you laugh over? Well that really depends, doesn't it? You can laugh about anything you like, on the inside. There is usually a quirky side to even the most traumatic of experiences. As long as you do not offend others, laugh as much as you like about anything you like. But the simple key is not to offend. So when involving others in your laughter, take care that the joke is for all. This is where your Emotional Intelligence skills will have to be good.

Having given yourself permission and understanding the importance of being aware of others' sensitivity, can you learn to laugh more?

Of course, you just need to look at life from different angles or seek out amusing material.

- ✦ Read comics and other humorous material.
- ✦ Choose to watch comedies instead of drama and tragedy.
- ✦ Spend more time with children.

- Pull faces in the mirror.
- Try to understand why others are laughing.
- Collect everyday anecdotes of life turned to laughter.
- Share embarrassing moments with others.
- Use toys and clothes to encourage humour.
- Give others permission to be amused and amusing.
- Forgive others for laughing in areas where you are sensitive.
- Remember everything can be funny if looked at from a different angle (but it doesn't mean you should necessarily laugh out loud).

For when all else fails in life and the stakes seem grim, at the worst of times when laughter appears furthest from your mind, remember the words of Victor Frankl from his experience of the Nazi concentration camps, backed up by the modern-day chuckle of cancer patients as the Clown Doctors entertain the oncology ward.

'I never would have made it if I could not have laughed; it lifted me momentarily out of this horrible situation enough to make it liveable.'

So you can chuckle at the tragic dance of life and hopefully come out on top. But don't forget you also have other alternatives for expressing spontaneous joy.

Why not dance?

Or even sing, to get you on the 'bright side of life'?

Or, where others are willing, enjoy wholeheartedly the pleasures of physical intimacy?

For laughter, singing, and dancing, along with the sensual experiences of intimacy, belong to primitive forms of Mindbody expression that allow you to achieve an innate 'flow' regardless of any necessary skill, as long as you are simply prepared to **Let Go and Be.**

Furthermore, these forms of expression blend all aspects of the primitive Mindbody, melding the physical, emotional and spiritual to the exclusion of the intellect, an all too rare achievement in the modern day. These are natural forms of physical activity that remain acceptable today and are often easier to apply yourself to than more formalised exercise regimes.

So why don't you enjoy these healthy forms of primitive expression more often?

Again, for most, it comes down to permission. Permission simply to let go and be with the rhythm. In the moment. You don't have to be with others (well at least for singing and dancing). No-one needs to see you. No-one, including yourself, needs to judge you, although in the case of physical intimacy you will need to take care in your choice of partners, so that this will be the case.

The more you can free up your mind and allow the inherent flow of the primitive Mindbody to absorb you, the more likely it is that you will be able to experience moments of personal release from the pressures of the modern intellectual world. This is not a condemnation of that world. You need your intellect as much as your creative side of Being, your rational left brain as much as your spontaneous right brain. Once again, we are simply highlighting the necessity of balance in our lives. It is likely that your intellect is already dominating your Being simply by living in a world that overwhelmingly focuses on doing instead of being. So it is time to allow your creative Mindbody to express itself instead.

For it is so easily forgotten that **We are Human Beings, not Human Doings!**

Why do you enjoy singing in the shower? Why do people enjoy karaoke? Or turning up the music in the car (how easy it is to think nobody is watching)? Or singing into the vacuum cleaner nozzle?

Because it feels good, natural. A part of your flow. No matter how good or bad you are at singing. Whatever else is happening in life. Because the flow of air is the flow of life's energy, as is the flow of your limbs and the beating of drums.

So give yourself permission, whether it be within the security of your own home, or out before the world, upon the stage. Reconnect with your primitive expression. Sing out loud. Dance the beat. Explore the pleasures of your intimate body. For, to put it simply, this is a vital part of you. A part that self-consciousness can too easily take away. And when you do allow this to happen to your Self, you simply lose so much more of life.

So how do you choose to express your Self today?

7

Learning to Be

Much of life is spent racing around on a stress-filled crusade to fulfil an endless set of self-imposed missions. Get the work done, time for exercise, get the children off to school.

But how much time do you set aside to just Be?

Being time, as opposed to Doing time, is very important. Being time is time set aside to relax and let the world go by. Release the day's tensions and stress, take a breath and recuperate. It should not be mistaken for pleasure time or time left for your life's passions, otherwise you will be short-changing yourself. Being time is time to empty your mind of all but relaxing thoughts, and allow the rest of your body to switch off for a period. It is time, therefore, that should involve no physical action, and only restful states of mind.

How do you feel about the suggestion of taking 20 minutes out of your day to download and get back to the inner reality of the fundamental You? Does it bring out a long deep release of breath? Does it feel good? It should. But if you are sitting there counting how many 'things to do' you are going to lose out of your day in doing this, guess what? You are a person who really needs to learn to relax.

Simply put, it is necessary to take time out in your day to relax, otherwise the stress of life is most definitely going to overtake you.

You should be trying to get at least 20 minutes of relaxation time during the day on a regular basis in order to touch base with your inner calm, and just Be.

Some individuals cannot possibly conceive of spending 20 minutes 'not doing anything'. If this is you, then start with five minutes and build every day by a little more. There are many different ways to bring your Self to a state of relaxation. As with most health related topics, the art of simply Being can become rather complicated, complete with scripts, tapes and metaphysical formulae. But here are a few suggestions that need no explanation. Try to find what works for you, so you can relax and reach a state of calm once or twice per day. Devoid of commitments, free of work, simply to Be.

Listen to Soft Music. Gentle, calming music is an effective way of reaching a state of calm. The key to what type of music you choose is not whether you like it or not, but the intensity of the beat. Choose forms of music that naturally settle your heart rate, which include Classical, Gregorian Chant, and most New Age styles.

Lie on Your Back and Watch the Clouds. No clouds? Then simply allow your Self to be absorbed into the deep blue above. Any natural environment, particularly in which there is a slow flow or absorbing depth, will bring a state of calm to your being. The sea, wind through the trees, and natural watercourses are examples of surrounds that will help absorb you into your inner being.

Daydream. Take yourself on a journey to a place of calm, be it real or imagined. Absorb yourself in a cocoon of warmth or relive the most relaxing and joyous moment of your life, allowing a smile to overwhelm your being.

Soak in the bath. Use bath salts, candles, aromatherapy, low light, music. It need not be a luxury, the only cost is in time (baths actually use up less water than moderate length showers).

Get a massage. Given a protective environment, you will feel the therapist take away the tensions of your body, while you allow your mind to simply unwind and drift away.

Meditation or Prayer. Meditation as a practice of focus doesn't need be associated with religion to create relaxing effects, so it is worth a try.

8

Goodnight, Sweetheart

How do you feel when you don't get enough sleep?

Tired, fatigued, unable to focus, irritable and with a decreased sense of wellbeing.

And the effect on your life, your work performance, your relationships, your health?

Not good, to say the least.

So once more we have a simple health truth. You need a good night's sleep. You don't need to know exactly what sleep does for your immune system, your stress levels, your muscle's ability to recover from physical exercise or your risk of depression. Sleep is simply critical to all these health factors and more, and you're yet again living in denial if you need an expert to convince you.

You know you need quality sleep and you know the effects of not getting it.

So what are you doing about it?

Chances are, most readers will answer, what can I do about it?

And the answer is, plenty, if you just think about how you live your life in relation to sleep. Consider how the following plan of action might improve your sleep and whether or not you can institute these simple actions for better sleep.

- First of all establish an appropriate time to go to bed on most nights of the week. Five out of seven nights would be a good start, allowing you to still enjoy the occasional night out. You will need to first consider how many hours of sleep you most feel comfortable with, which can vary between people (but is usually between six and nine hours). Then set your ritual hours in bed.

Be prepared to adjust these time frames if you get it wrong.

- Prepare for bed. Wind down over the hour or two before sleep. Do not activate your mind with study. Do not 'adrenalise' your mind with action television. Do not stress your mind with the late breaking news that rarely affects you directly, but may leave you overwhelmingly concerned about the state of the world.
- Once you're in bed use it for what it is intended for. Sleep. Or activities that may lead to sleep. These are few and far between. A good book or classical music. No study, no high level discussions, no arguments—unless you intend them only for the sake of having an excuse to physically make up!
- Ensure you get enough exercise during the day to use up your energy stores, but don't exercise too close to sleep. The gap between exercise and sleep is for you to decide, but it needs to be satisfactory enough to allow the body to return to less activated states of being than are present during exercise.
- Create an environment for sleep. If you live in the city make certain you can darken your room and eliminate night noises. Otherwise you will be on a constant state of alert at every sound that enters your room.
- Make your family and friends aware that you won't take any calls after your wind down time—unless it is an absolute emergency.
- If you sense you are feeling stressed towards your wind down time, start off with a relaxation technique.
- Make sure your room is not too warm or too cold. Either extreme of temperature will limit your ability to get to sleep.
- Remove the alarm clock (if you need one) to a place where it is not visible.
- If you use an electric blanket to warm your bed, turn it off once you are in the bed. Leaving it on will dehydrate you, and you may also be sensitive to the electromagnetic forces. Some individuals are also very sensitive to outdoor power boxes near their bedrooms.
- Go to the toilet before going to sleep to avoid night waking. Avoid alcohol, coffee, tea or large volumes of fluid before bed.

These are simple means to creating an environment pertinent to sleep. Have you tried to institute such changes to your life to improve your sleep?

If not, now is your chance.

Here are a few more suggestions to consider if changing your environment does not do the trick. They involve foods and medications (further pertinent information including Nutritional Supplementation is covered in Section 5).

- Consume moderate levels of protein in your diet. If you eat according to the plan in this book you will be doing this. Why is this important? Proteins supply the amino acids from which your brain's neurotransmitters are formed. And you can't have a balanced brain without healthy neurotransmitters. Among the neurotransmitters required for healthy brain function is the hormone melatonin, which is essential in governing our wake and sleep patterns (see Section 5, Chapter 8, 'Neurotransmitter Health', for tips on how to maintain healthy melatonin levels).
- Balance your energy intake so that you avoid peaks and dips in your blood sugar levels. Once again, the eating plan in this book will help you do this by focusing on complex carbohydrates with a steady release of energy during digestion. Avoiding high carbohydrate foods before and after dinner is also recommended.
- Do not use stimulants, especially before bed. Stimulant-containing substances include cigarettes, caffeine, soft drinks with caffeine (e.g. colas, energy drinks), alcohol and recreational drugs. Even if recreational drugs help you get to sleep, the state of sleep you achieve will not be complete, leading to later sleep disturbances.
- If you suspect a medication you are taking is interfering with your sleep, ask your doctor to review your prescription.

Lastly, there are many medical conditions that can affect your sleep. If all else fails, seek advice from a doctor, or referral to a Sleep Clinic. A life without sleep is a life drained of energy, vibrancy and happiness.

You simply can't deny it.

SECTION 3

Forget Dieting, Simply Choose Healthy Eating

Do not be mistaken. Few, if any, fad diets work in the long-term. What in effect happens to most addicted dieters is a constant bounce between dieting and binge eating, with little room in the middle for sensible moderation. Any diet which requires you to force yourself into a restricted eating pattern will only last as long as you can maintain a psychological fortress of constraint against your primary emotional drives. Furthermore, the gains from any diet will not last if the body's own inherent needs that cause you to be hungry in the first place are not addressed. What we are suggesting is simple common sense eating, the natural way, for the rest of your life.

Following the basic premise, everything in moderation as long as it is natural, healthy and cooked sensibly. Without any pressure, fault or failure if there are little luxury indulgences on the side.

Keeping it simple, keeping it natural ...

With one simple specific dietary intervention that may ultimately change how you feel, as well as shed kilograms from your weight. And that is an understanding of your own personal Food Intolerances and their effect on your health and wellbeing. We strongly recommend that you participate in a Food Elimination Regime as outlined in Chapters 6 and 7, in order to increase your awareness of your body's personal food intolerances. In our experience, the lesson learnt in individualising your eating habits can be literally revolutionary in terms of your health, happiness and weight control.

1

Understanding Your Hunger

There is a simplistic view of dieting that suggests that losing weight comes down to the net difference between the energy you consume and the energy you burn. Eat less, work more, and the kilograms will be shed. Very simple, hardly sexy, and if left to this very basic formula, not necessarily a recipe for healthy living.

Other approaches might complicate matters a little by throwing in the terms high carb, low fat, or high protein, and in so doing appear to render a diet acceptable, as long as energy in is less than energy out.

Yet, is this acceptable?

No. Why?

Because the human body has far more complex nutritional needs than simple energy maintenance. The argument that energy in versus energy out is all that should matter to weight loss is ridiculous. If a person's healthy caloric intake (a measure of the energy they consume) was 2000 calories, and that person consumed 2000 calories of sugar or any other food in isolation (substitute a single vegetable, meat or fruit if you like), nobody would argue that they are not going to be healthy, let alone alive, for very long! No rocket science required here.

Energy balance is not all there is to consider when looking at what we eat. We have complex needs, even if simple health guidelines can help us attain them.

So what are our body's needs from food?

Balanced Energy Intake: Yes, it is important, but not the be all and end all. Energy supply is primarily derived from our intake of carbohydrates, with additional supply from fats. Proteins may also supply energy, but this is not necessary or preferable.

Building Blocks for Spare Parts: Want to repair your body from the damage normal life is inflicting on your muscles and organs? You had better feed it quality protein. Want to build a better body? More protein. To keep your cellular membranes flexible, think essential fatty acids. Doesn't matter how much energy you get from your carbohydrates, they won't replace proteins and healthy fats in the latters' role as fundamental building blocks for the body.

Do we need to get more technical than this? Hopefully not, because it is certainly obvious that your car needs more than just a full petrol tank. And if you don't give it regular maintenance with replacement parts it is not going to get far. Want a bigger, better, faster car? More basic building blocks required. Same with your body. It needs quality proteins and essential fatty acids if you are going to have a quality body for your carbohydrates to fuel.

Nutrients: Think of vitamins, minerals and a complex array of other natural chemical chains as lubricants to your body's biochemical reactions. You might have the parts, you may have the petrol, but if you don't have the glue or the match to bind your parts or ignite your energy, work doesn't happen as it should. So we need a long list of vitamins and minerals as much as we need energy and protein to make us work. So much so that we will crave some of them, just as we crave to improve our energy.

Fluid: Water is the most important element in the working of the body. It is the river of life required for all other actions of our body. Without it we are no more. Simple. That is why we thirst, and sometimes, that is why we hunger, too, for unfortunately many of our body's natural urges are not as accurately related to our body's needs as we would assume.

Now let us consider the basic human organism for a moment. Let's make it more simple still and forget for a moment its higher faculties; its intellect and emotions. Put it to work in feeding itself for optimal performance, driven only by its physiological needs, without regard for emotional eating and rationalised diet programmes.

Given this, what would such a being reflexively hunger for?
Only to meet its energy intake?
No, because it could consume all the energy it wanted and still fail to

thrive without protein to repair muscles, or nutrients to aid this repair. And without fluids, it would be lost even sooner.

Logically it would hunger for energy, but also proteins, essential amino acids, nutrients and water.

And that is what the human organism does, before our brains get in the way.

Wait a moment, you are saying, my hunger drive doesn't tell me what to do. It just tells me to eat. Not exactly true. You do crave foods, don't you?

Most of you would answer 'Yes, but chips, chocolate and soft drink aren't healthy. And that is what I crave'.

True, but you are still craving something.

Problem is, modern society has derailed the link between what we crave and what we actually get.

Smart man has fooled himself. With artificial foods, flavours, textures, fillers. And even when we eat a healthy meal our modern food combinations make it hard for the body to accurately obtain what it wants. Here are a few practical examples of what we mean:

- ✦ Have you ever craved fatty, deep-fried chips? Cheese and butter? Healthy? Not exactly. But when your body wants fat, this is what it now relates to. What might your body actually be craving? Potentially it is craving the essential fatty acids found in deep water fish, nuts and seeds, avocados and so forth.
- ✦ Craving a steak? You may need the nutrient iron (particularly for menstruating women) or protein (for people undertaking hard work or exercise). But what else might you unfortunately get if you follow this urge continuously? A high level of saturated fat if you choose the wrong cut and do not remove the fat. The result, a meaningful craving becomes a potential health risk.
- ✦ What about CHOCOLATE? Perhaps you are looking for an increase in your magnesium levels, and chocolate is the strongest environmental stimulus that parallels your body's natural quest for magnesium.

- Sweet biscuits, cakes, soft drinks, candy—this list is endless. These foods are also the quick fix to low energy, brain fatigue and tiredness, the problem being a quick bounce back to the depths of a sugar low several hours later. Unfortunately again, the body naturally chases the strongest associated stimulus with the food need it desires, which is no longer necessarily the healthiest choice. Whole fruits, vegetables, legumes and pulses consumed with a protein source would provide a more balanced return of blood sugar stability.

- Perhaps you are just hungry, with no particular craving? Have you tried drinking first? Maybe you are actually thirsty. Try drinking first and see what happens to your food craving, for our thirst and hunger response are not always clearly defined.

Do any of these cravings appear familiar? The reality is, hunger is a 'fuzzy' sensation, particularly now that we have modified so many of our foods. Hunger is a message, but we have scrambled the codes in artificial flavours and foods cooked in vastly complex ways, so much so that we have painted over the codebook needed to decipher the message.

Remember, we haven't even taken into consideration that we have lopped off our heads and discarded our minds for the moment. And, as with many things human, removing the brain doesn't necessarily imply making matters worse. Not when it comes to eating. Bring back the brain and we suddenly add emotional eating and dumb logic into the equation (the fact that there is a 'beer diet' is all the argument you need to prove the latter).

So all we can now say is this. If you're hungry it implies your body needs at least one, but more than likely a combination, of the following:

- A boost of energy from carbohydrates
- More building blocks in the form of quality protein or essential fatty acids
- Vital nutrients
- And/ or fluid (good advice is to drink first, ask questions later; a certain way to decrease your calorie intake!)

If it could communicate better, your body would probably be screaming:

'And all of these in healthy forms please! No sugar bounces, few saturated fatty acids, forget the additives, the colourings and if you can afford it, go organic.'

There is a simple message here. Respect your hunger. Don't ignore it. It is telling you something. You body wants 'something' healthy to eat. So however well or badly you read your body, the least you can do is eat healthily, regardless of how cloudy your vision is as to what in particular your body may need. This we will need to work on a little more, once we've replaced your lopped off head cleansed of complicated ideas. For we need to understand how to optimally achieve each of the four body needs above (along with a fifth concern, adequate fibre intake) if we are to carefully work with our hunger drive in a healthy manner. Focus on one issue such as energy control at your peril, for this is how you will create a well-meaning but unintentionally unhealthy diet that in the long term will not sustain any weight loss it has achieved. Your body can't maintain weight loss in a diet state; instead it simply wants to survive!

It is important to understand that many fad diets have serious health implications, including:

- Diets that cause malnourishment and nutritional deficiencies along with the sought after weight loss, through low protein and nutrient intake resulting in medical complications, fatigue and so forth.
- Diets that eventuate in weight rebound as soon as the body is given the opportunity to recover its protein and nutrient sources. The rebound comes with the eventual return to the diet of fats and sugars as the body quests for the protein and nutrients it has missed. This occurs in 90 per cent or more of fad dieters within a year.
- Symptoms such as fatigue and vagueness from low carbohydrate intake on a very low energy diet, however high the protein levels consumed in an attempt to compensate for this.

You need to match all of the needs of your body for food, not just energy balance, if you are to eat well. And if your goal is to lose weight, this is just as important, because there will not be any long-term weight loss if all of these needs are not met. You will simply crave food and eventually consume it, in a search to restore adequate energy, protein, essential fatty acids, quality nutrients and/ or sufficient fluid intake that was deprived during the period of your dieting.

Note we are emphasising **sustained long-term weight loss** here. Most fad diets that you can survive in the short-term will lose you weight. But what is the point if you simply can't sustain it?

2

A Quick Look at Energy Balance

We have already mentioned the simplistic interpretation of classic 'dieting' in terms of energy consumption, and argued strongly that while energy balance is important, it is not the only issue that needs to be focused on. But we will take a moment to look at this issue in more detail, if only to highlight how concentrating on a single diet concept often becomes more complicated than is necessary to simply shop and eat.

The level of our body's energy intake combined with the breakdown of energy stored as body fat needs to be adequate to match the energy we expend during daily activity. No energy, no fuel, and the many motors in our body start to wind down. Starve yourself and they stop; it gets no simpler than that. If we consume too much energy we will store it as body fat, whether it be eaten in the form of carbohydrate, protein or fat, for the body transforms each of these into its conventional storage unit, body fat. And this is how we literally get 'fat' as we store more and more energy as a result of our excess energy consumption.

On the other hand, if we consume too little energy we will burn body fat in order to make up the shortfall. This is how we lose the body fat we are currently storing. Unless, of course, we have inadequate energy stores, we've taken dieting too far or we're malnourished to begin with, in which case we will break down our other body constituents, suffer from fatigue and the overall body dysfunction that is associated with starvation.

Our primary and preferred source of energy comes from carbohydrates; from the breakdown of the sugars found in cereals and grains, legumes and pulses, fruits, vegetables, and dairy products. We may also burn animal fats and the oils present in vegetables. Finally, although less preferable, we can utilise protein as a source of energy if required.

But we predominantly use carbohydrates as our short-term source of fuel. The complexity of the energy issue comes from this, for in being a short-term source of fuel, the utilisation of carbohydrates is complicated by the need to keep our blood sugar levels relatively stable throughout the day. We must balance the rise in our blood sugar levels after a meal with the falls that will occur as we use energy through normal body function, or more dramatically, during exercise.

This is no different to your car. Flood the engine with too much fuel and the motor won't work properly despite having fuel. Why? Because too much fuel is not a good thing. This is true for the body as well. Flood your body with sugar and your body starts to dysfunction. In the short-term the body may compensate for this state, but over the long-term, disorders arise due to the effect of high blood sugar levels on the rest of the body, leading to Diabetes Mellitus (Type 2) and its complications and associated conditions grouped commonly under the daunting title of 'Syndrome X'.

On the other hand, allow your blood sugar levels to drop by not eating enough high energy foods and your engine also begins to falter. In modern society this rarely leads to starvation and energy crisis, however, because your body's own defences combined with a food rich environment means this won't happen unless you are wilfully (and inappropriately) starving yourself through diet. Instead, your body will throw off a set of signals (hunger, cravings, light-headedness, headaches, clouded thought, visual disturbances, nausea, mild body shakes) encouraging you to act on the matter. Eat something, anything, that is energy rich.

Bring me carbohydrate rich foods! Bring me biscuits, chips, pasta, sweets, DONUTS! NOW OR ELSE!

So there you have it, the swings and falls of outrageous carbohydrate cravings and the effects they have on your body!

What does this equate to in food terms?

The practical implication of trying to balance your blood sugar levels is the need to make sensible food choices when it comes to consuming from the carbohydrate group. This implies understanding the effects of the foods you eat upon your body. Some foods load your body with sugars rapidly and others do so in a more controlled manner. Interestingly, those foods that contribute to rapidly build up your blood sugar levels in the short-term (one to two hours) also drop the blood sugar below normal levels soon after, thus becoming a double-edged sword. You get hungry again, eat more, and repeat the process in a series of high and low blood sugar swings.

How do you know what foods these are? First of all, they will only be foods from the carbohydrate containing food groups; meat, fish and eggs do not have carbohydrates in them. After which, you can look at a scientific measure known as the Glycemic Index (GI), a measure of the rate of sugar uptake that will result from consuming a food. You will also need to consider how much of the food you are going to eat, known as the Glycemic Load. Eating a little of a high GI food, for example a single sugary sweet, may change your blood sugar level far less than a big bowl of pasta, even if the latter's GI is considerably lower.

Why? Because there is far less sugar in the sweet than in the big bowl of pasta, despite the slower rate at which the pasta enters the system. In other words, pouring very little fuel into your tank very quickly is going to have less of an effect than pouring a lot of fuel in slowly. There's just not enough sugar in one lolly to make a dramatic difference!

Getting complicated, isn't it? Particularly when you realise that foods you think are quite similar often have a different Glycemic Index. You thought rice was rice, but that isn't so. You now need to know which rice is nice, and which is less than nice to your blood sugar level—and in what quantity!

Can you be healthy without this level of information?

Is the stress of working it all out going to kill you instead?

Don't panic! If you like all the mathematics and table searches there are plenty of books out there on the Glycemic Index. And every time you have lunch you can do the sums, keep your GI as low as you can and see if it works for you (but don't forget to look at the Glycemic Index AND the serving size, or read the newer tables on Glycemic Load that combines your Glycemic Index and serving size for you, providing you with a new number to work with).

Or you can take a step back and say, 'It's got to be simpler than this'. After all, monkeys do it without textbooks.

Well, yes. That is the point of this book. So let us think less in terms of dietary labels and simply consider the food we eat in terms of how you would buy it from the supermarket. When we look at a food on the shelf or in the fridge, what does it mean to us? Not just in terms of energy and Glycemic Index, but protein and nutrient value, fibre and fluid intake.

Let's just call a food a food and get on with it.

So what was the point of this chapter?

Simply to show you that we can get deeper and deeper into theories and labels, values and tables, until we're totally confused and afraid to enjoy food. Which works well for diet creators because they can always find a new way to create a new table and a list of recipes to fill another book. For if you are not measuring Glycemic Index and Glycemic Load, then you could count calories, balance zones, lower fats or carbohydrates, measure protein, vitamins and minerals, fibre count, or take into account magic nutrient numbers, physiological and biochemical lists, body and blood types and so forth.

Forget it. Keep it simple.

See a food for what it is and go from there.

For simple is sexy. Or at least by spending less time on the mathematics of dieting you can spend more time on ... well, that's your choice. ☺

3

Understanding What You Eat

Let's learn a little about the actual foods we eat. From this we shall derive some easily followed health rules that we can apply to creating a Healthy Eating Plan. Note that the following are general rules that should always be adapted or modified if you discover you have individual food intolerances (see Chapters 6 and 7) or other health requirements.

Meat, Poultry, Fish and Eggs provide the protein that builds our essential body. Adequate protein levels are therefore essential to healthy life maintenance. Eating protein is also vitally important in reducing our hunger. Finally, vital nutrients including iron, zinc and Vitamin B12 are derived from animal forms of protein, without which there is a risk of inadequate intake unless carefully accounted for.

The major concern regarding this group of foods, however, is the associated fat content. With a little care such concerns can be minimised by following these guidelines:

Red Meat

Choose lean and heart-smart varieties of red meat (beef, veal, lamb, pork). Remove all visible fat. Do not consume processed meats other than as a savoury treat for they are very high in fats and nitrates.

> *Consume lean red meat at least twice per week for it is high in iron, zinc and Vitamin B12. A commonly used and simple guide to serving size is a cut of red meat equivalent to the length and thickness of the palm of your hand.*

Poultry

Poultry is a low fat source of protein if the skin is removed. Concern is often raised regarding the antibiotics administered to growing poultry, so where possible choose organic chicken.

Eat at least one or two serves of poultry per week. Organic is preferable. A commonly used guide to serving size is a palm and half a finger's length of chicken, with skin removed.

Fish and other Seafood

Two serves of deep water oily fish (salmon, ocean trout, sardines, herring, tuna and mackerel) per week is excellent in providing the omega-3 fatty acids critical to almost all cellular function, due partly to its vital role in the formation of all cell membranes as well as in the brain. Leave the skin on fish for it contains much of the oil you are seeking.

BUT unfortunately there is a catch. Consuming such fish puts you at risk of high toxin (mercury, dioxin, PCB's, pesticide) levels that may also be detrimental to your health. The larger the individual fish eaten, the greater the risk due to the accumulation of toxins in predatory fish.

A maximum of one serve of larger individual fish (a filleted or steak style serving) per week from the large fish families (tuna, ocean trout, salmon, mackerel) is therefore recommended. Canned fish is generally safe in the quantities suggested as a can is supposedly derived from numerous smaller fish, but if you eat more than three serves per week, beware of the source!

All other seafood and fresh water fish contain low to moderate levels of Omega-3 fatty acids, and also represent excellent protein sources. The bottom line is, eating fish and/or shellfish is a healthy and important component in the human diet. **But again, be wary of swordfish, shark (flake) and other large individual fish sources.**

Aim for at least three serves of fish per week, with at least one serve of deep sea oily fish. A commonly used guide to serving size is a fish fillet or single steak style cut to the size of your hand.

Eggs

Eggs are an excellent protein source for most people, but as with many food choices there exists a subgroup of people for whom eggs are not the best choice. These people experience an increase in cholesterol from egg consumption. If you know you have high cholesterol, restrict your consumption of eggs to one to two per week. Otherwise a higher egg intake (three to four eggs per week) may be consumed, but it is recommended that you review your cholesterol levels three months later. Lastly, eat eggs in a runny form, that is, raw, poached or soft boiled, for prolonged heat may denature the oils and proteins.

Vegetables

Non-starchy vegetables should represent more than half your plate at lunch and dinner (and breakfast as well, if you are able to adjust to this style of eating). Vegetables are an excellent source of nutrients, fluid and fibre. They also provide for the slow release of carbohydrates. Furthermore, when eaten raw or lightly steamed they require significant chewing prior to swallowing, an action that lessens the hunger response independent of the amount of food consumed.

The most important quality of vegetables, however, is their nutrient value. Along with the better known nutrients such as the vitamin and mineral groups, vegetables also contain a multitude of additional phytonutrients (complex plant based nutrients) whose health benefits are continually being discovered. Each vegetable type is comprised of a different set of vitamins, minerals and phytonutrients, so the greatest health gains in the area of nutrient intake come from consuming as much and as many different vegetables as possible. The importance of this to your health cannot be overstated.

Do not fear, you cannot overeat from this food group (to be absolutely certain of quality, eat organic).

> *Consume as many servings of vegetables (except for potato, sweet potato and corn) as possible. This means at least two cups at each main meal. Steam them, salad them, soup them but just serve them and eat as much as possible, no questions asked. In other words, more than 50 per cent of your plate should be taken up with vegetables in as many different colours*

and varieties as possible. And while you are at it, throw in an unlimited variety of fresh herbs and spices for both flavour and nutrient value.

Fruits

Fruits provide similar benefits to vegetables in terms of nutrient intake, fibre and fluids. They also contain a higher concentration of carbohydrates, but if eaten whole, most fruits do not significantly elevate blood sugar levels, thus being excellent energy foods. As with vegetables, fruits are high in different vitamins, minerals and phytonutrients, so you should consume as many different varieties as possible to maximise your nutrient intake. While there are some exceptions, fruit is generally a healthy food group to be strongly encouraged.

Aim for two to four serves of fruit per day. Don't overdo the tropical fruits, however; keep to half a banana, a medium sized mango, one passionfruit or kiwi fruit, or a few dates. Nor should you over consume fruit juice. Keep this for drinking during main meals only, no more than a cup once or sometimes twice per day. As for dried fruits, include minimal amounts only for they are concentrated forms of sugar intake.

Nuts and Seeds

Eaten in moderation, nuts and seeds are an excellent source of quality proteins, healthy fats and various vitamins and minerals. They are an excellent grazing food, ideal for reducing between-meal hunger. Variety again is the key, for different nuts and seeds contain different nutrient values. Nuts and seeds should be eaten raw, not roasted or salted.

A small palm-full of nuts and seeds are also an energy dense, protein rich, essential fatty acid mix. A good snack choice.

Legumes and Pulses

Legumes and pulses, otherwise known as beans, are the highest source of fibre available, as well as providing controlled carbohydrate release. Similar to all natural food choices, they again provide vital vitamins, minerals and phytonutrients. Do we need to repeat that you should consume as many different varieties as frequently as possible?

Eat at least a serve a day of cooked legumes, pulses or beans, each serve equalling approximately a half cup. They are not absolutely necessary, but a very healthy option in addition to vegetables for added fibre and nutrients, and definitely a preferable option to serves from the cereal/ grain group. They may also be used to substitute for a protein serve if you do not wish to eat meat or fish (use one cup in this case).

Starches

The starch foods—cereals, grains and starchy vegetables (potato, sweet potato and corn)—include the high carbohydrate foods modern society consumes in abundance. These foods have been built into the modern food pyramid on the assumption that humankind needs high levels of cereals and grains to function.

This is an interesting argument, since for all but the last 10,000 years of human evolution man did not grow the crops from which cereals and grains are derived. In fact, many societies did not have access to these crops at all until colonisation, and it is interesting to note that these very same peoples (e.g. Australian Aborigines) are also the same communities that struggle most with diet related diseases such as Diabetes Mellitus (Type 2) in modern society. As for the starch vegetables, again, these were not available to most of the human population until the advent of sea travel to the New World, the natural home of potato and corn. So the modern emphasis on cereals and grain groups, to the extent represented by many high carbohydrate diets, is a little confusing to say the very least.

So where did we once get our energy from? A higher fat diet with a healthier range of fats (more fish, and red meats from leaner breeds that had to run away from predators). From a range of gathered legumes, nuts and seeds. And from a higher fruit and vegetable intake. And we managed to do this without cereals and grains, despite having a greater energy requirement (there were few sedentary jobs in the Stone Age!)

The human species is not dependent upon the cereal/grain group to be healthy for there is enough carbohydrate and nutrient (vitamins and minerals) coverage in all other food groups for our energy requirements IF we consume a balanced diet containing a high intake of fruits, vegetables, legumes, nuts and seeds.

Foods from the cereal/grain group do have their place (the exception being those with Coeliac Disease or Food Intolerances to cereals/grains), but certainly not to the extent emphasised in the Western diet.

Cereals and grains can remain a healthy addition to a diet when consumed in complex form, that is, where little processing has taken place prior to eating. But most of our grain-based foods come to us processed; white or wholemeal rather than wholegrain breads, white rice, processed breakfast cereals and pastas, cakes, biscuits, muffins, donuts.

And the result? Fast release and/or high carbohydrate density foods with little nutrient value (destroyed by the processing), which also usually require additional oil or sugar based substances for flavour. Remember, it's not just the food you eat but what you use to flavour it that adds up the calories so be aware of what you spread on your bread, the nature of your pasta sauce, the chocolate coating on your biscuit etc.

Therefore, if you want to eat from the grain group you should look to wholegrain foods such as wholegrain breads, pastas and brown rice. Please note, however, that there is a myriad of non-conventional cereals and grains such as quinoa and amaranth that are far better for you than most conventional cereals. One meal which has trained us to eat cereals is breakfast, and here we suggest a natural rolled oats based muesli or porridge rather than heavily processed commercial cereals or toasted breads.

Which brings us to an important point. One of the main problems with consuming from the cereal/ grain group is that it often means simply eating wheat, and occasionally rice. The problem with this is that wheat is a food that many people find hard to digest (we shall discuss 'Food Intolerance' in an upcoming chapter).

A more sensible choice would therefore be, yet again, to vary the type of cereals and grains eaten. Rather than just eating wheat, consider a daily and weekly mix of cereal and grain sources that also includes rice, barley, oats, rye, amaranth, quinoa, millet, polenta or buckwheat. Such a range of cereal and grain consumption will yet again provide you with a high and varied nutrient intake directing you towards healthy living.

As for the starchy vegetables; potato, sweet potato and sweet corn are healthy foods when taken in moderation (and when not deep-fried!). They provide for excellent nutrient and fibre intake, but unfortunately carry a high and relatively hastily released concentration of carbohydrates. Eat them in the moderation recommended and they remain an enjoyable and healthy part of your diet.

> **No more than three serves daily in total from the cooked starchy vegetables group: squash, corn, potatoes, sweet potatoes (one serve equalling a moderate sized potato or a cob of corn)**
> **OR**
> **three serves from the cereal/ grain group: breakfast cereals (a serve being half a cup of cereal), breads (one slice), cooked pasta or rice (a serve being half a cup)**
> **OR**
> **Three serves daily in total as a combination of both food groups.**

You may have two serves at breakfast since you may require additional energy early in the day. It is preferable to have your remaining serve at lunch rather than dinner for similar reasons.
Remember, all measures of volume are taken when cooked.
Using uncooked volume as a guide is certain to lead to overeating. See end of chapter for serving size measures.

IN OUR EXPERIENCE WE FIND THAT THOSE INDIVIDUALS WHO CHOOSE TO LIMIT THEIR SERVES OF THIS GROUP ARE IN FACT MUCH HEALTHIER AND HAPPIER.

Dairy

Dairy as a nutrition source beyond the age of infancy is controversial (and uniquely human). For a start, human milk has multiple differences from cow's or goat's milk. Many people are therefore unable to digest animal milk products satisfactorily, leading to food intolerances due to the lactose and casein proteins found in such products. And while dairy does contain high levels of calcium, population studies show little consistency between the amount of dairy consumed and the risk of osteoporosis, the condition for which dairy consumption is usually encouraged.

Fermented forms of milk, the predominant variety of which is yoghurt, are the preferred source of dairy, as the fermentation process partially breaks down milk protein, as well as adding vital gut-friendly bacteria to the diet. As long as you are consuming the level of dairy we are recommending, go full-cream, and enjoy it!

Dairy is usually tolerated by most people if consumed in moderation (3/4 to one cup per day). We therefore consider it to be an optional food if consumed in these moderate amounts unless a Food Elimination Regime identifies that you have an intolerance to it.

Fluids

We should all be ensuring we get plenty of fluids; 6–8 glasses of filtered water per day. Many of us try, many also fail. Don't worry if you are among the latter; our eating plan has a safety catch. If you consume the levels of meat and fish (as long as not over cooked), fruit, vegetables, legumes/pulses, and cereals/grains in whole form, you will be consuming a high level of fluid even before raising a glass. But still raise the glass as often as possible to ensure adequate hydration.

Consume 6 to 8 glasses of water per day.

Alcohol, Tea and Coffee

Alcohol in moderation is acceptable as there are beneficial effects to limited consumption. But there is a fine line between moderation and over consumption, so be diligent in keeping your alcohol intake to two standard drinks per day. The same rule applies for Tea and Coffee. You can read more on this in Chapter 11 of this section, 'Drink and Be Merry'.

Restrict your alcohol, coffee and tea to two standard drinks of each per day.

Spreads, Oils, Dressings and Sauces

These are useful in encouraging healthy eating if you apply them in moderation over healthy meals. But the key is moderation. The healthiest choice is cold pressed extra virgin organic olive oil which can be lightly drizzled over salads or spread over bread in the Mediterranean fashion. Another useful oil dressing is a mix of vinegar, lemon and fresh herbs.

Commercial spreads, dressings and sauces are not recommended as they are often high in both salt and/ or sugar.

The arguments over butter versus margarine are likely to continue as long as advertisers are well paid to do so. However, the key question rarely asked is, how often are you needing a spread on your bread? Spreads become less of a concern if you do not overly focus on bread as a staple in your diet and do not lavishly apply any spread you use.

> Use salad dressings, sauces and spreads in moderation. It is preferable to make your own salad dressings using extra virgin cold pressed olive oil, vinegar, lemon juice and herbs.

Processed Foods

In this section we are considering the processed foods you are purchasing at the supermarket, including bread, commercial breakfast cereals, pastas, canned soups, sauces and dressings, confectionaries and potato crisps—the list is endless. We are considering these foods within the context of purchasing from the supermarket as part of your ongoing diet, as opposed to pleasure foods purchased as a treat.

Any food that is processed has had its quality changed, and rarely for the better. Yes, it may be more edible, but that does not equate to being healthier. Nutrients are extracted, proteins and fats denatured with a long list of preservatives, colourings and other additives. Within processed foods there are a whole plethora of chemicals the body is not necessarily built to effectively manage. Even 'natural' food isolates that have been processed arrive in our gastrointestinal systems in a form so altered that the body struggles to adjust.

Every processed food is different and the body's ability to manage these foods depends on the level of processing and types of additives involved. Ideally, therefore, we recommend, wherever possible, avoiding processed foods. It's probably the only way to keep it simple, short of suggesting you take a three-year course in food processing to understand what they are literally doing to our foods at the bakery, the breakfast cereal factory, the soup kitchen, biscuit company and so on.

FORGET DIETING, SIMPLY CHOOSE HEALTHY EATING

If you are undertaking this Healthy Food Plan with a wholehearted commitment there is little need to be attracted towards processed foods found in your supermarket for the following reasons:

- Most processed foods other than those canned for storage purposes (fruit, vegetables and beans) are in the cereal/ grain group (biscuits, breakfast cereals, pasta, potato crisps, confectionaries, pre-cooked meals) and are hence limited by this Healthy Eating Plan.
- Since you will no longer need to purchase these foods in the quantities you previously have been, we strongly recommend making your own where possible (homemade biscuits, breads and pastas within the limitations of your cereal/ grain serving number and sizes).
- The simple and healthy cooking methods we are suggesting should mean meals are not too time consuming to prepare (salads, steaming, smoothies, soups, stir-frying, grills). In which case there should be no need to purchase pre-prepared, pre-cooked or frozen meals (including canned soups).
- Otherwise these foods represent pleasure foods (biscuits, cakes, potato chips, confectionaries) and should only be consumed as a limited treat. In which case you should be buying quality not quantity.

Avoid processed foods wherever possible. Wherever possible make homemade alternatives from healthy recipes, always accounting for appropriate serving number and volume.

Salt

Given that you are following the above Healthy Eating Plan, a small pinch of Salt on your meals should not be of concern. The only exception is a subgroup of people with hypertension who are considered salt sensitive, because their blood pressure elevates with salt consumption. However, this does not inclulde everybody with high blood pressure, and therefore you might want to discuss this with your doctor if you have problems with your blood pressure before altering your dietary salt intake.

Increased salt intake can creep into your diet without direct use of salt if you eat processed foods. For instance, most commercial soups are high in salt. There are other areas to be aware of if you have a concern regarding your salt intake:

- Soy, tomato, sweet chilli and similar sauces
- Canned legumes (bean mixes)
- Canned vegetables

If you are going to use canned goods (and here we mean canned ingredients such as legumes, vegetables or fruits rather than heavily processed foods) in a limited amount, it is sensible to decide which are likely to be the most practical for your kitchen. For instance, we find the limited use of canned foods most practical when it comes to canned legumes that otherwise require soaking and cooking before use, while we seldom use canned vegetables other than artichokes and water chestnuts.

Sugar

As for Sugar, we recommend removing added sugar from your day whenever possible. It is our experience that most people feel far better after removing sugar from their diet. The reality is, the moment you consume most processed foods such as biscuits, cakes, soft drinks and confectionary you are consuming a large quantity of added sugar. And it may come as a surprise but there is even more natural sugar in your fruit juice and that supposedly healthy fruit muffin as well. Finally, look out for canned fruits and most sauces, as they too contain large servings of sugar.

For this reason you do not need to add even more sugar to your diet than is already sneaking in, in hidden forms. Nor do we recommend using any artificial sweeteners as these are often linked to food intolerances. You may experience a short-term adjustment in your taste before feeling completely comfortable with a no added sugar diet (one to two months). But eventually you will gain from the added flavours you begin to notice in natural foods that are otherwise blunted by the overpowering sweetness of sugar.

Pleasure Foods

And lastly, the Pleasure Foods and Party Meals. Life is about getting it 95 per cent right and enjoying whatever else comes your way, and the same is true of eating. As long as you are not going out of your way to find the 5 per cent that is wrong about your diet and making it 20 per cent!

Therefore an occasional pleasure of a small sized quality treat with a meal is not going to destroy your health unless you have particular dietary limitations (e.g. food allergies, extreme intolerances). But make it small and make it quality. A single scoop of gelato rather than four scoops of cheap ice cream. A connoisseur's quality chocolate treat rather than a bar or multiple blocks of supermarket junk. After all, one healthy snack we know falls into the pleasure foods category is a small quantity of dark chocolate per day, known to have antioxidant benefits.

Yes, it makes your mouth water, doesn't it? So enjoy treats occasionally, abiding by the simple rules. Make it occasionally, and go quality, not quantity.

The occasional meal dined out on rich indulgent foods is not going to kill you either. Two or three meals out of the 21 in a week is an acceptable celebration of life, as long as it stays at this level. The key is ensuring you are aware enough to retain your week by week eating plan, rather than becoming paranoid about your meal by meal food intake.

Ninety per cent commitment is enough if you are genuine. Two to three quality indulgent meals per week and the occasional treat in between should be enjoyed guilt free!

4

Creating a Healthy Plate

If we put these rules together and bring it back to the simplest way to understand food, what you put on your plate, what does it look like? Here is a simplified example of the range of options available to you with this eating approach, **remembering that you need to adapt your own plan to any personal Food Intolerances (see Chapters 6 and 7).**

BREAKFAST

UNBREAKABLE RULE: To be healthy in the long-term you must eat breakfast!

1. 1–2 serves of oat based muesli with additional nuts and seeds mixed in with ⅓ serve of milk and/ or ⅓ serve of natural yoghurt. Mixed fresh fruit—½ banana, strawberries, kiwi fruit, apricots, pears etc.
2. Try some grilled zucchini, mushrooms and tomato with dried herbs and toast (if not having muesli), avocado (if not having as a snack) and a soft (runny) boiled egg or some beans.
3. Similarly, try grilled vegetables served with piece of meat, healthy sausages or fish.
4. Omelette with vegetables, a single serve of toast with fruit.
5. A fruit smoothie with a mix of fruits, water or milk, nuts, protein powder if you are taking it (more on this later), blended through to the consistency you are comfortable drinking.

6. A large fruit salad with a serve of natural yoghurt.
7. A winter porridge from oats with a fresh fruit serving on the side.

We advise starting your day with a glass of warm water with lemon juice. This helps regulate your bowels and gets you in the habit of increased daily fluid intake.

Additionally you can include a herbal tea (such as green tea) or your usual tea/coffee with milk as desired.

SNACKS

1. Handful of nuts and seeds
2. A piece of fruit

LUNCH

1. An unlimited quantity of salad/vegetables with an appropriate serving size protein source (fish/meat/chicken/legumes).
2. Non-starch vegetable and/or legume/bean based soups. This might also have meat or fish in it (e.g. laksa), with or without an open single slice of bread or unflavoured rice/corn cracker.
3. Sushi or a healthy Asian stir-fry.
4. As long as you are accounting for your starch vegetable servings carefully, why not try a single jacket potato with a bean salad dressing and a fresh vegetable salad serve on the side.

DINNER

1. What about a stir-fry with meat, poultry or seafood? Add a serving of rice if you have cereal/grain servings in reserve.
2. Steamed fish with steamed vegetables.
3. Grilled meat or fish with grilled vegetables and a side salad.
4. A chilli con carne with beans and minced meat, limit the rice.

DESSERT

1. Fresh or stewed fruit for 'dessert'.
2. A single treat of quality chocolate.

Now, do you think you can eat this much? If not, remove the cereal/grain serve from any meal. It is not essential. It is there to provide you with added energy, but if you have low activity levels this may not be needed. Do not force yourself to eat more than your fill, simply leave food on your plate, and that food should be from the cereal/ grain group. Chances are you have put too much on your plate to start with if you are serving up pasta or rice, due to the expansion that takes place during cooking. Remember, serving size is by cooked volume, not raw volume.

There are a few groups who may need to modify their general eating plan for their own personal requirements. They will fall into either of two groups as follows:

People with Low Energy Requirements
If your activity levels are restricted due to physical incapacity:

- If you have diagnosed Insulin Resistance or Diabetes Mellitus.
- If despite all arguments, you are going to put yourself on a calorie restricted diet.
- If you have undiagnosed low metabolism such as may be present with Hypothyroidism.

If this applies to you, remove the cereal/grain group from your diet. These foods are not necessary. You could also restrict your fruit intake to two fruits per day. But do not alter your protein, vegetable or legume/ pulse (beans) consumption for they will provide you with necessary protein, energy and nutrients.

People with High Energy Requirements (Athletes)
If you are an athlete, exercise intensely or do hard physical labour you may need to increase your energy intake. The traditional argument is to increase your carbohydrate levels, which has usually been interpreted

simply as more cereals. Truth of the matter is, cereals and grains will provide more energy. But if you are exercising intensely you need more than just energy. You will need more building blocks to both repair the damage on your body and make it stronger. That means more protein. And you will need more nutrients in order to strengthen your immune and detoxification organs as well. And that means fruit and vegetables along with the given protein.

So if you need more from your eating plan than the average person, increase your food intake in sensible proportions. Bigger servings of all groups; meats and fish, eggs, fruit and vegetables, wholegrain cereals and bread. Then watch your weight and ensure it does not rise. Assuming you are as hard working as you believe, this is unlikely to happen unless you lessen your intensity of training and maintain your high energy/ nutrient/ protein diet. In which case step down your food intake as well.

Of course, another group of people with high energy requirements include women who are pregnant or breast-feeding. In either case, we recommend the series of books by Francesca Naish and Jan Roberts, such as *Better Pregnancy* and *Better Breast-Feeding*, as thorough discussions of required nutrient intake are beyond the scope of this book.

Relevant Serving Sizes to Consider

Remember you can have unlimited quantities of vegetables (non-starch), fruits (non-tropical, fresh) and legumes (beans, chickpeas, lentils etc) every day!

RED MEAT (Beef, Lamb, Pork)
Palm size thickness cut.

POULTRY
Palm and half-finger size cut.

SEAFOOD (Fish, Shellfish)
Hand size fillet or serving.

STARCHES
Cereals/Grains/Pasta

Bran cereals, flaked	½ cup
Bran cereals, concentrated	⅓ cup
Dry oats	¼ cup
Puffed cereal	1½ cups
Shredded wheat	½ cup
Other unsweetened cereals	¾ cup
Cooked cereals	½ cup
Bulgur (cooked)	½ cup
Pasta/noodles (cooked)	½ cup
Rice (cooked)	½ cup
Wheatgerm	3 tablespoons
Taco shells	2

Bread (per slice, 30g/1oz)

All Breads	1 slice
Pita	½
Bagel	½
English muffin	½
Plain roll, small	1
Tortilla (30cm/12ins across)	1
Rice/corn cakes	2–4

Crackers

Rye crisps	4
Wheat crackers	2–4
Rice crackers	8–10

Pastry

Biscuits	1
Plain muffin, small	1
Pancake (20cm/8ins diameter)	2
Waffle	1

STARCH VEGETABLES

Corn on cob	1
Corn by cup	½ cup
Baked potato (small)	1
Mashed potato	½ cup
Yam, sweet potato	⅓ cup

TROPICAL FRUITS

Banana	½
Figs	2
Honeydew/Rockmelon	⅛ melon
Mango	1 moderate size
Papaya	1 cup
Pineapple	¾ cup, ⅓ can
Watermelon	1¼ cup
Avocado	½

DAIRY/ SOY MILK

1 cup non fat, skim or whole milk
½ cup concentrated skim milk
200g yoghurt
1 cup soy milk

FOOD VARIETY IN SNACKS AND DESSERTS

Fruits
Stone Fruits: Apricot, Peach, Nectarine, Plum, Cherries, Apple, Pear
Citrus: Orange, Mandarin, Grapefruit, Tangerine, Lime
Tropicals: (Limit serving Sizes) Banana, Melon, Pawpaw, Guava, Lychee, Star Fruit, Mango, Pineapple, Kiwi Fruit, Passionfruit, Coconut
Berries: Raspberry, Strawberry, Blueberry, Blackberry, Logan Berry, Cranberries
Grapes and Currants
Avocado

Nuts
Almond, Brazil, Cashew, Hazelnut, Peanut, Pecan, Pine, Pistachio, Walnut

Seeds
Pumpkin seed, Sesame seed, Sunflower seed

Dairy (if tolerant)
Yoghurt, Ice Cream

Carob or Quality Dark Chocolate

Refreshments
Filtered or Mineral Water
Milk (limit as per dairy), Coffee, Tea (preferably Herbal)
Alcohol (limit servings)
Blended Fruits (preferable to limited juicing) or Fruit Smoothies

VARIETY OF THE MAIN PLATE (LUNCH/DINNER)

ANIMAL PROTEINS:
Red Meats: Beef, Lamb, Pork, Veal, Game (Rabbit, Kangaroo etc)
Poultry: Chicken, Turkey, Duck
Deep Sea Oily Fish: Tuna, Salmon, Herring, Mackerel, Sardines
Other Fish (Fresh or Salt)
Other Seafood: Prawns, Mussels, Lobster, Squid, Octopus, Oysters, Scallops, Crab, Bugs
Eggs
Protein Powder

FATS:
Olive Oil, Margarine, Butter

LEGUMES/PULSES:
Green beans, Snow and Snapped peas, Adzuki beans, Black beans, Bean curd, Black eyed beans, Borlotti beans, Cannelini beans, Chickpeas, Fava, Gabunzo, Haricot, Kidney beans, Lentils, Lima beans, Lupins, Pinto beans, Soya beans

FAT

MEATS

STARCHES and/or LEGUMES

STARCHES:
MAX. 3 SERVES/DAY

Cereals/Grains:
Amarunth, Barley, Buckwheat, Bulgur, Millet, Oats, Quinoa, Rice (Various varieties), Rye, Sagoa, Semolina, Spelt, Tapioca, Triticale, Wheat

IN THE FORM OF:
Pasta, Breakfast Cereals, Breads, Noodles, Muffins, Cakes etc.
OR
Starch Vegetables:
Potatoes (Different varieties), Sweet Potatoes, Corn, Parsnip

LIMIT SERVING SIZES

VEGETABLES
Choose as wide a variety as possible from the following types

Leafy Greens:
Spinach, Cabbage, Silverbeet, Pak Choy, Bok Choy, Wombok, Lettuce (Varieties), Rocket, Chicory, Endive

Mushrooms:
(All Varieties)

Sea Vegetables:
Seaweed

Root Vegetables:
Carrots, Beetroot, Garlic, Ginger, Radish, Water Chestnut

Marrows: Cucumber, Eggplant, Pumpkin, Squash, Zucchini

Fresh Herbs: Coriander, Basil, Dill, Marjoram, Oregano, Turmeric, Fennel, Watercress, Bay, Cardamom, Cinnamon, Fenugreek, Mint, Rosemary, Thyme, Tarragon, Parsley

Brassicas: Brussel Sprouts, Broccoli, Cauliflower

Stalks: Celery, Asparagus, Leeks

Others: Tomatoes, Onions, Celeriac, Capsicum, Chilli, Artichoke

5

Enjoying Your Healthy Eating Plan

The simple meal examples in the last chapter gave you an idea of the meal options available to you. But let us dedicate a chapter to a more comprehensive look at the meals you can make on this program. After all, what is on your plate is going to be the primary determinant of whether or not you will commit to a Healthy Eating Plan over the long term. Rather than give you exact recipes to follow over a pre-set period, we shall provide you with a meal preparation guide, and allow you to choose what flavours you wish to use (see Sauces, Marinades, Rubs).

The meals suggested have been categorised according to meal time (Breakfast, Snacks, Lunch, Dinner, Dessert) and cooking type. An important health rule when it comes to diet is to choose a healthy and simple cooking style. The healthy cooking styles suggested involve minimal food processing and hence are also quick to make:

1. Fresh foods presented either as Salads, Natural Breakfast Cereals or Fruits Salads
2. Fruit Smoothies
3. Soups
4. Steaming
5. Stir-Frying with minimal oil or with water only
6. Grills
7. Roasts and Casseroles.

From the above list you should choose on a daily basis:

1. Three Main Meals per day: Breakfast, Lunch and Dinner
2. Marinades, Sauces, Dressings and Rubs as required for these meals
3. Snacks (one to two per day) with an optional healthy dessert with your main evening meal
4. Adequate and regular fluids.

Otherwise the predominant rules from the last chapters are built into the meal guides, these being easily summarised as:

1. Respect serving numbers for the day especially in regards to the cereal/grain, starch vegetables and dairy groups
2. Respect serving sizes for these groups
3. Use natural ingredients, not processed foods.

Note that both Lunch and Dinner come under the title of Mains. This is because the meals you choose are interchangeable and what you choose usually depends upon lifestyle. In fact there is no reason why you cannot eat Main meals for Breakfast either, other than cultural habit. We do not, however, suggest interchanging Breakfast suggestions for Mains other than for Grills.

Breakfast

There is a most important rule that pertains to breakfast in particular. You may have noticed it in the previous chapter, but it bears repeating:

UNBREAKABLE RULE: TO BE HEALTHY IN THE LONG-TERM YOU MUST EAT BREAKFAST!

Countless studies have shown the importance of a meal in the morning on health and performance. This applies regardless of what is eaten. Now we would prefer you to be eating a healthy breakfast, preferably with a protein source, because people really do feel and think much better in the morning for it. But the first step if you are one of those on the go people whose habit is to chug down a coffee to get you through to mid-morning or lunch is to have anything solid! As you'll see from the following breakfast suggestions, a healthy breakfast will take you no more time than an unhealthy one to make.

A healthy breakfast does not comprise several pieces of toast, or of the much-advertised highly processed breakfast cereals, often held together with sugars and other odds and ends. Breakfast should comprise of a diversity of foods, preferably including fruits, nuts, seeds and a source of protein such as eggs, yoghurt, meat or fish. This does not mean every breakfast must contain all these food groups, but a mix throughout is preferable. One thing to note is that many people report feeling much better after starting a breakfast with a protein serve in it, despite their initial reluctance to do so. All we can say is, give it a try.

There are three general choices for a healthy breakfast; a muesli based natural breakfast cereal, a smoothie or a hot breakfast. While a breakfast cereal is the common choice of many in Western society, this is probably due more to ease of preparation rather than any other reason. Indeed the recent swing towards high protein dietary approaches have swayed many towards having a quality protein source at breakfast. The fact is, your lifestyle may dictate what you eat for breakfast as much as anything else. Choosing any of the three suggested options are healthy approaches to breakfast as long as balanced with the remainder of the day.

Any breakfast at all is better than no breakfast.

Cereals

As long as it's balanced with your intake for the rest of the day, a breakfast cereal can be a healthy option. If you choose the right cereal! Forget highly processed 'wonder' cereals commercially advertised by sports players, who may (although this is unlikely) need nine serves a day in order to achieve the energy necessary for their out of the ordinary high workloads. Your choice should instead consist of:

1. Oats based muesli, whether fresh or as porridge. Remember to account for your cereal/grain group servings if you make this choice. One cup of muesli or porridge oats will generally equate to two serves, leaving you one serving of cereal grain for either lunch

(preferably) or dinner. This is not a bad option for using your cereal/grain servings. After all, they provide you with vital nutrients and energy at the best time of the day, in the morning, just before you get active. On the other hand, dinner servings of high energy cereal/grain foods will not be utilised, and may instead be stored, leading to weight gain.

Therefore, in terms of your three cereal/grain/starch vegetable servings, a two serving breakfast, one serving lunch, and no servings dinner is a good approach.

2. ½ cup of dairy as either milk or yoghurt for your muesli or porridge. This allows for the remainder of your day's dairy to be used in coffee, tea, or perhaps over a fruit dessert.
3. Any fruit desired over your cereal, with the only limit being a single serving of tropical fruits at any one sitting (mango, ½ banana, kiwi fruit etc).
4. Nuts, seeds, freshly ground LSA, lecithin and/or psyllium husks may also be added to your cereal. A mix of these will give you an additional serve of nutrients and fibre.
5. Fresh water or, less preferably, a fruit juice with your meal.
6. Coffee or tea, if you so choose.

This should generally suffice for breakfast for most people, reinforced by a healthy snack choice as a mid morning meal, unless you are competing in sport or have a heavy physical workload.

Smoothie:

Here's your alternative quick start breakfast. All you need is a food processor or blender. And if you want to get fancy, a book on fresh juicing. With smoothies, the aim is to keep as much fibre as you can tolerate from your fruits (preferably all) and add more ingredients.

1. Choose any fruit (although generally not citrus as this group curdles). Try a wide variety throughout the week. Careful not to

overuse the tropical fruits, although a ½ banana serve is useful in creating a creamy texture for those who do not wish to add dairy. Try various combinations. Create your own flavours or reproduce from a juicing book.

2. Add ½ cup of milk or yoghurt if you do not have dairy intolerances. This generally works with most fruits (other than citrus).
3. Nuts can also be added in small, and preferably mixed quantities (the food processor will grind the nuts if left to blend a little longer).
4. Eggs or protein powders will add a protein serve to the mix without generally affecting taste, a good way to get a small to moderate protein serve when you're not happy with meats in the morning.
5. Filtered water can thin out your smoothie if you do not like a creamy consistency.
6. Most supplements (including probiotics) can be added to a smoothie if they can generally be taken with food. Tablets may be pre-broken in a coffee grinder. Note, however, that fish oils and flavoured supplement powders may alter the taste of smoothies.

Juices

Juicing can be helpful in providing you with additional nutrients, somewhat like a supercharged multi-vitamin. But this comes with a concentrated dose of sugars. Although the sugar from a single serve of fruit may not elevate your blood sugar levels all that much, the number of fruits used to extract a single juice means the total load may lead to a greatly increased intake of energy (in fact many juices have more sugar in them than a can of your favourite sugar-laden soft drink).

Furthermore, much of the sugar in fruit comes in the form of fructose. While this has the benefit of limiting the blood sugar rise that occurs with a serve of fruit, a growing number of people are demonstrating fructose intolerance, possibly due to our general increase in juice intake. Interestingly, fructose is a volume related food intolerance, meaning that to control its irritations, a person unfortunately needs to restrict intake across a wide variety of fruit and vegetables. Professional assistance is certainly required here.

What then to do about juicing? Firstly, vegetable juices consumed with meals are healthy food choices, as they do not carry with them the sugar content of fruit juices. But start adding additional fruits and the following considerations need to be taken into account. If you choose fruit juices, juice yourself and immediately before food consumption, and drink with main meals.

1. If you are going to have a citrus or other juice, return as much of the pulped fibre as you can tolerate. Preferably water it down by ½ or ¼ concentration.
2. Diluting does not generally apply to vegetable juicing, which contains far lower concentrations of sugar.
3. Consider combining vegetables and fruit to overcome some of the less favoured flavours of vegetable juices.
4. Consider the use of herbs for flavour as well as medicinal reasons, such as garlic, ginger, mint and parsley.

Hot breakfasts

1. One or two eggs (poached, boiled, lightly scrambled, frittata or quiche) make a healthy protein alternative to red meat, chicken or fish.
2. Unlimited addition of non-starch vegetables. Grilled vegetables such as mushrooms, capsicum, onions, zucchini and eggplant can be flavoured with fresh herbs and leafy green vegetables (unlimited quantities).
3. 1-2 serves of wholemeal toast may be added in the morning as long as accounted for in your day's cereal/grain serves (and intolerances to wheat or other cereals/grains do not exist).
4. If you do not use your dairy serves elsewhere, consider a small(!) amount of grilled cheese for flavour.
5. Alternatively, choose a grill (see over page).

Mains

Most main meal recipes remain viable options in our Healthy Eating Plan if consumed with respect to volume. Ironically, when we review the food approaches of most imported cuisines (Asian, Italian, Indian), we find healthy recipes that have been distorted through volume exaggeration (pasta, rice, and, in some instances meat servings), while vegetable content has been drastically diminished. The simple solution is to enjoy the same foods with the food groups re-proportioned.

Grills (for any meal)

Grilling food is an option for any meal of the day. Use olive oil if necessary, but keep it to a minimum or apply by basting brush.

1. A serve of meat, fish or poultry. Follow the hand rule discussed previously as a guide to serving size.
2. A grill and salad combination makes a perfect lunch or dinner. If you need to eat more to be satisfied, begin with a vegetable-based soup.
3. Away from breakfast, boiled or roasted starch vegetables such as corn (one cob) or potato/sweet potato (moderate single potato size) can be added to your grill provided you do not exceed the combined cereal/grain and starch vegetable limits for the day.
4. Similarly, grilled (or roasted) vegetables may be added to a small(!) serving of pasta in the traditional Italian style, drizzled over with a herb infused olive oil (and don't forget to leave a small amount of dairy serve for the parmesan cheese). Consume as a side dish or entree to grill and salad, not as a main.

Sauces, Marinades, Rubs

These are ways to add extra flavours to your meals. If you keep what you add to a minimum it may not matter that much what you choose. Drown your foods in flavouring, and that's a different matter.

1. Be careful with commercial sauces and marinades which are usually full of sugar, oil and/or salt. Make your own instead.

Use recipes founded on olive oil, yoghurt, vinegar, lemon juice, crushed tomato or reduced stock as your base where ever possible. Add an assortment of fresh herbs and dried spices. Look out for added sugar. Use honey in preference, but also in moderation (yes, it's natural, but so is sugar).

2. Have you thought of a rub? No, we're not suggesting a massage, although they're nice, aren't they? A mix of herbs and dried spices rubbed onto meat, chicken, fish or shellfish, prior to being grilled or otherwise cooked. Straight herbs and spices without the added oil. All in all a very healthy flavouring option.

3. Use lemon to bring out the flavour of your foods prior to eating. A touch of salt will also help, and for most, is not harmful, if eating an otherwise healthy diet.

Salads

Salads are an excellent source of high nutrient value foods. The only guarantee that your foods will remain the powerhouses of nutrients expected of them is when they are eaten fresh, whole and raw. A salad a day is an abundant supply of vitamins, minerals and phytonutrients. Make it a protein salad with the addition of egg, sliced beef, chicken pieces or fish.

1. All non-starch vegetables can be tossed into your salads without concern. The only limit in your choice is your taste and imagination.
2. Fruit can make a tantalising addition to many salads (grapes, citrus, berries, mango, avocado …) Again, your imagination or willingness to find new recipes is the only limit.
3. Many exotic salads also include a mix of nuts and seeds.
4. Potato, sweet potato or corn kernels may also be added, but respect serving sizes.
5. A salad can be turned into a complete meal through the addition of red meat, chicken, fish and shellfish (appropriate serving sizes), beans and sensible volumes of pasta or rice. Meat and fish can be added as a warm or cold salad, whatever your preference.
6. Dress with olive oil, vinegar, lemon and lime and an unlimited

number and variety of fresh herbs as desired. Use Asian style sauces (soy, oyster, fish, sweet chilli) or dairy based sauces (natural yoghurts, Caesar salad dressing) in moderate amounts only due to their sugar, salt and dairy content. Avoid commercial dressings as they are high in vegetable oils.

Soups

Soups are an easy way to consume a high intake of vegetables, while if you become more inventive, you can add all variety of foods; red meat, chicken, fish, beans and so forth. Soups should be homemade. Commercial soups are generally full of salt, vegetable oils and preservatives. An easy way to create a variety of soups through the week is to prepare a large amount of stock base (vegetable, chicken, beef or fish), freeze appropriate portion sizes, and add to different food combinations as you desire. Consider buying a insulated container to keep your soups warm at your workplace.

1. Use a freshly prepared stock base found in any basic recipe book, (vegetable, chicken, beef or fish).
2. Consider using all leafy greens for clear soups as well as the stalk vegetables (e.g. celery, leek).
3. Marrow, brassicas and root vegetables for winter style creamy soups are excellent warming foods (pumpkin, zucchini, squash, eggplant, broccoli, cauliflower, beetroot, turnip, carrot, onions).
4. Remember those fresh herbs (coriander, lemon grass, basil, oregano, mint, marjoram, garlic, ginger, thyme, tarragon, chilli) as well as spices (turmeric, saffron, cinnamon).
5. Chicken, beef, fish, seafoods or beans can be added to create a meal (e.g. laksa).
6. Be careful not to overdo it if adding noodles (in Asian style soups) or pasta (in minestrone). One serving size per person is generally enough, but all too often overestimated, leading to overeating.

Steaming

A quick, easy method of cooking which retains most key nutrients. Far preferable to boiling when it comes to vegetables (which tend to leach nutrients into the water).

1. Most vegetables can be steamed if cut into small enough pieces. Steaming retains most of the natural flavouring of vegetables. Preferred steaming vegetables include the leafy greens, carrots, cauliflower, broccoli, cabbage, pumpkin, zucchini and squash.
2. Pre-soaked beans can be also heated by steaming.
3. To complete the meal, steam fish, creating a delightful tender meal to melt in your mouth. Flavour with a rub or lightly drizzled sauce. Fresh herbs should be put on after the steaming process is complete.
4. Steamed rice should be measured for volume when cooked. Remember the size of a serving is only ½ cup cooked, and you have limited servings in your day.

Stir-Frying

Asian style stir-frying using olive oil is also a healthy form of cooking, as long as you take care not to overcook. The key is to use minimal oil and to allow the steam to do much of the work. This is why a good wok is essential. A vast array of vegetables can be thrown in with herbs and spices to flavour the meal. Add in fresh herbs as close to completion as possible (or after the meal is on the plate) to retain the greatest flavour, avoiding the need for rich sauces. Lightly **pan-frying** larger pieces of meat or fish risks the overuse of oil, so take care in what you add. You can use water instead of oil.

1. All leafy greens, mushrooms, carrots, garlic, ginger, marrows (if shredded or sliced thinly enough), onion, tomatoes, capsicum and the brassicas can be stir-fried in whatever volume you want. You can also add beans and beans sprouts.
2. Shredded zucchini, carrot or other root vegetables can be used to replace noodles or pasta.

3. Add chicken, beef or other red meats, fish or shellfish in appropriate quantities. Beans and nuts may also be added for a change in flavour and texture.
4. Rice or noodles should be measured for volume if cooked. Remember the size of a serving is only ½ to ⅔ cup cooked, and you have limited servings in your day. This also applies if what you are stir-frying is being added to pastas or, indeed, toast.
5. Fresh herbs (coriander, basil, chilli) should generally be added in as late as possible to retain their flavour.

Roasting/Casseroles/Baking

As long as meals are not overcooked, roasting, baking and casseroles are a healthy option.

1. Ensure the cooking time is appropriately accounted for in regard to the weight of the meat or poultry you are roasting. Medium rare is a healthy cooking choice for roasting.
2. Fish baked in foil retains much of its juices, and is delicious when herbs and spices are added.
3. Do not over consume from the starch vegetable groups (potatoes, sweet potatoes), and keep volume size in relation to the day's serving of cereals/grains and fellow starch vegetables.
4. Look to roast a variety of other vegetables with the starch vegetables you normally use to make up the bulk (garlic, eggplant, pumpkin, squash, zucchini, onion, fennel, celeriac).
5. Serve on a fresh bed of leafy greens to add variety to the meal.

These should be your main cooking styles. Other styles should only be used on rare or special occasions. They are **barbecuing, baking (if only because you're likely to be baking cakes, pastry and biscuits) deep-frying and chargrilling** with the use of **rich sauces and dressings**. Better still, don't use these methods at home at all. Save them for eating out so that when you consume food from a cooking style that is less healthy, you're getting a quality treat.

Snacks

When you reach for a snack, the key question to ask yourself is are you really hungry or are you just craving a junk food? You know what a junk food is. There's either junk or food. No in-between.

Here is a guide to some healthy snack alternatives:

1. All fruits, as long as you are not over consuming from the tropical fruits group (½ banana, moderate mango or equivalent size of pawpaw)
2. Handful of seeds (pumpkin or sunflower)
3. Soups kept in a thermos (non-starch vegetable and/or legume/bean based soups)
4. Palm full of mixed nuts; walnuts, brazil, hazel, cashews, almonds, pecans (25g/1oz)
5. Fresh vegetable salad
6. Pieces of fresh celery, carrot, peppers with low/no oil dips (eg hummus)
7. 50g of fresh avocado with lemon and herbs
8. Herbal tea, usual tea/coffee with milk if desired

Dessert

Ah, dessert ... the delight of life for many an addicted soul.

1. If you have desserts regularly, focus upon whole fruits most days of the week.
2. Frappes—chilled, blended fruits—are a healthier alternative to flavoured ice creams and sorbets (which are often loaded with additional sugar).
3. For winter, consider stewing or baking fruits for a warming end to your meal.
4. Remember to consider your dairy servings if you are a dessert addict. This little extra delight may be the cause of your waistline.

But it may also be the cause of your happiness ... which one would hope will compensate a little for a few extra centimetres!
5. Break the pastry habit if you have one.
6. If you break the rules, go quality, not quantity e.g. a small piece of quality chocolate, noting that dark chocolate has antioxidant properties!

Fluids

First rule, keep well hydrated. Second rule, don't depend on coffee, tea, alcohol, fruit juice or soft drink to do the job. The key is:

1. Drink adequate amounts of filtered drinking water. This should amount to six to eight glasses per day.
2. All other forms of fluid intake should be limited to two servings per day. This includes fruit juices (which contain more sugar per serve than most soft drinks).
3. Eliminate soft drinks from your diet.
4. See smoothies for guidelines regarding their use.

Now look at the above cooking suggestions. We have two points to make here.

1) None of the above will take long periods of time to prepare. Remember the five simple cooking styles—Smoothies, Salads, Soups, Steaming and Stir-Frying (along with Grilling)—if you want quick, simple and healthy meals. Food should be enjoyed but unfortunately in this fast paced world a 'bite on the go' can often be a necessity, so remembering your quick healthy options is a must to retaining a Healthy Eating Plan.

This is particularly pertinent to breakfast and lunch. Make them easy food choices, particularly if you have a fast paced life. Otherwise the takeout meal is going to be far too hard to ignore.

2) You don't need a long line of recipes telling you what to eat on every day over the next eight weeks. As long as you are choosing from a long list of nutritious foods that you are not intolerant to, balance out your meals sensibly, and cook in a healthy manner, you will be creating healthy delicious meals. By all means look for tasty recipes on a meal-by-meal basis, but there is no secret on Day 3 Week 2 of your healthy eating plan that isn't going to work on Day 6 of week 8, or in 10 years' time!

The reality is, most of us eat in a relatively repetitive manner anyway. We are simpletons, having a basic array of meals we fall back on time and time again. So here is a suggestion. Think of these basic meals in terms of the cooking methods you are going to use to cook your primary protein source, and just vary the ingredients according to the wide range of different foods that can be cooked by this method.

6

The Quest for Magical Foods

Now, we have talked about food groups in general and the relative balance between their intake.

But what of specific foods?

Are there any truly magical foods that you just must eat?

Well here are a few suggestions from a mix of sources:

Beef for protein, iron, zinc and B12 ... oysters for zinc and making love ... salmon, tuna, herring, sardines, ocean trout for omega-3 oils ... seaweed for iodine ...

Avocados are full of good fats, an apple a day keeps the doctor away and apricots make you live longer, just ask the Hunza.

Beans, beans and more beans for fibre and a multitude of phytonutrients, be they azuki, black-eyed, kidney, pinto or cannellini. Or other legumes such as lentils, lupins or chickpeas. And soy because it is full of isoflavones and phytoestrogens, theorised to reduce the incidence of breast cancer in Japanese women. Better eat them too, whether or not you are Japanese (soy beans, not Japanese women).

Blueberries save your brain, bananas for natural potassium, then there is celery, a natural diuretic and carrots for beta-carotene ...

You can go nuts on nuts and get a sea of amino acids, vitamins and minerals depending upon whether you choose almonds, brazil, cashews, hazelnut, macadamia, pecan, pistachio, peanut or walnuts ...

And the same from your cereals and grains depending on your choice of amaranth, barley, corn, oats and rye, a little bit of wheat or try tapioca.

Pears are high in boron, prunes keep you regular, and pumpkins are high in antioxidants such as lutein and zeaxanthins (must be good!).

There are foods that will give you lots of lycopenes (such as tomatoes), quercetin (such as onions) and whole host of sulphur containing foods to support your liver detoxification pathways (like artichoke, broccoli, cabbage and cauliflower). And don't forget leafy greens are high in Vitamin K too.

Since there are thousands of useful phytonutrients, there is likely to be a parallel list of fruits, vegetables, nuts, legumes, cereals, and weeds that are also magical, because they contain the highest percentage of one or other exotic but healthy plant compounds. That is why you should eat lots of different herbs as well; coriander, turmeric, garlic, ginger, cinnamon, chilli ...

There are as many different 'sexy' foods as there are sexual positions in the karma sutra (including some positions that involve foods). Dark chocolate and wine are also great, and they're sexy, too!

And 101 different juicing combinations including every fruit, vegetable and edible grass.

And let's not forget the humble zucchini just because it sits at the end of the culinary alphabet, or mushrooms because they sit in the dark and are fed ...

They're both good for something too!

Do you get the point of this?

Our point is that most natural foods contain nutrients beneficial to our health. Is that surprising? Of course not, that is why our body eats this selection of foods in the first place, and not tree branches, lawn grass and coral.

Because they are good for us.

The search for a magical food is interesting but overlooks the simple fact that we need so many different nutrients from so many different foods. What would happen if you decided to eat a concentration of one particular food? Let us say, carrots. Wonderful, eat lots of carrots. Obviously, however, after eating lots of carrots, you won't have as much space to eat from another food group, which may have equally valuable health benefits. This, and you may turn a little orange, but that's another story.

So you can focus on a particular food claim for a specific problem to a certain degree, but ultimately you will still need a whole list of nutrients from a diversity of foods to remain healthy (a further chapter on this particular aspect of Magical Foods later).

Furthermore, have you checked out the magical food claim? Does it stand up to scientific reasoning? And are you eating the magical food in the particular manner in which it provides you health benefits? And without potential side effects? Might you be eating too much of it, so much so that the magic food becomes a tragic food?

Eating a quantity of food is OK to a point, but the more you eat the more you risk overburdening your digestive system with a single food, hence leading to possible food intolerances and other potential gut responses.

Moderate red meat intake, wonderful. Excess meat intake, increased risk of constipation, calcium depletion and several types of cancer.

Increased oily fish intake from salmon, tuna or ocean trout, wonderful. Get your Omega-3 fatty acids in. But without taking into consideration the risk of mercury toxicity from eating large deep water prey fish, a risk.

Consuming increased quantities of soy has also been questioned due to the fact that modern soy extraction and processing is very different to the traditional manner of soy consumption found in Japanese culture. Maybe traditional forms of fermented soy found in Japanese style soy products aid in reducing breast cancer risk, but do soy products and extracts created by the rapid production techniques utilised in modern society have the same effect? Or no effect at all? Or do they make matters worse?

Only time will tell. So what do we advocate?

If you hear of a magic food and are confident in the claims made regarding it, fair enough. But only consume it within the overall balance of your overall Healthy Eating Plan. We suggest no more than one portion of any single food per day, two maximum. Instead, eat from a wide variety of foods to optimise your intake of a diversity of nutrients. This will also have the additional benefit of protecting you against developing food intolerances (which we shall discuss in detail in the next chapter).

The following is a table of high nutrient foods. Note that every nutrient in this table is essential for good health; the outcome of reading this table should be an increased awareness of why eating a diversity of foods is essential to maintaining good health.

HIGH NUTRIENT FOODS

ESSENTIAL MACRONUTRIENTS	
Essential Amino Acids	Animal Meats (Fish, Chicken, Liver, Beef, Pork, Veal) Nuts, Seeds, Beans (incl Soy beans), Dairy, Eggs
Omega-3 Fats	Deep Sea Oily Fish—Salmon, Tuna, Herring, Mackerel Other Seafood, Avocado, Nuts and Seeds
Fibre	Beans, Whole Fruit and Vegetables (incl Potatoes) Whole Grains, Nuts and Seeds

VITAMINS	
Vitamin A	Cod Liver Oil, Carrots, Sweet Potatoes, Squash, Spinach, Beetroot Leaves, Broccoli, Parsley, Chives, Watercress
Vitamin B1	Nuts (Pine, Peanut, Pistachio, Brazil), Seeds (Sesame, Sunflower), Oats, Wheat, Buckwheat, Egg Yolk
Vitamin B2	Liver, Nuts (Almonds, Cashews), Mushrooms Legumes (Soybeans, Lentils, Mung), Avocado Asparagus, Leafy Greens, Broccoli, Egg Yolk Millet, Rye
Vitamin B3	Animal Meats (Fish, Chicken, Liver, Beef, Pork, Veal) Bran, Mushrooms, Brown Rice
Vitamin B5	Liver, Eggs, Beans (Soybeans, Peas) Whole Grains, Mushrooms Leafy Green Vegetables, Broccoli
Vitamin B6	Animal Meats (Fish, Chicken, Liver, Beef, Pork, Veal) Beans and Lentils, Brown Rice Nuts (Hazelnuts), Whole Grains (Rye, Barley, Wheat) Avocado, Bananas, Potato, Sweet Potato Spinach, Brussels Sprouts, Leeks
Vitamin B12	Animal Meats (Fish, Chicken, Liver, Beef, Pork, Veal)
Biotin	Brown Rice, Liver Soybeans, Bean Sprouts, Peanuts, Wholegrain cereals

Folate	Liver, Beans, Leafy Green Vegetables, Lettuce, Spinach, Broccoli, Lentils, Nuts
Vitamin C	Peppers, Broccoli, Brussels Sprouts, Cauliflower Cabbage family, Strawberries, Raspberries, Blackcurrants Tropical Fruits (Guava, Pineapple, Honeydew, Kiwi, Mango), Turnips, Squash, Radishes Asparagus, Citrus fruit (Oranges), Parsley, Spinach, Watercress
Vitamin D	Fish liver, Milk, Egg yolk
Vitamin E	Beef, Nuts (Almonds), Seeds Sprouts, Egg yolk, Leafy Green Vegetables, Whole Grains
Vitamin K	Broccoli, Cabbage, Lettuce, Spinach, Soy beans Liver, Pork
ADDITIONAL NUTRIENTS/NUTRIENT SUPPORT	
Choline	Lecithin, Beans, Liver, Egg Yolk, Milk, Green Leafy Vegetables
Inositol	Lecithin, Beans, Whole Grains, Nuts and Seeds, Milk
Carotenoids	Wide Variety of Coloured Vegetables
Bioflavinoids	Fresh Fruit and Vegetables generally Apples, Oranges, Peaches Berries (Blueberries, Strawberries) Currants and Grapes, Tomato, Onions Parsley, Sage, Red Wine
Coenzyme Q10	Animal Meats (Fish, Chicken, Liver, Beef, Pork, Veal) Nuts, Seeds, Beans (Soybeans)
Carnitine	Animal Meats
Lipoic Acid	Liver
Lactobacillus	Fermented Dairy (Yoghurt, Kefir), Miso, Tempeh

MINERALS	
Calcium	Dairy, Nuts and Seeds (Almonds, Walnuts, Pecans) Green and Dried Beans, Lentils Leafy Green Vegetables, Spinach, Broccoli, Cauliflower Brown Rice, Whole Grain Wheat, Corn Citrus Fruit, Avocado, Artichoke, Garlic, Onions, Bananas Root Vegetables (Beetroot, Turnip, Carrots, Squash)
Magnesium	Nuts and Seeds (Almonds, Pecans, Cashews, Walnuts,) Green Peas and Dried Beans, Lentils Whole Grains (Wheat, Rye), Corn Leafy Green Vegetables, Spinach, Broccoli, Cauliflower Brown Rice, Citrus Fruit, Figs, Avocado, Artichoke, Garlic, Onions, Celery, Bananas, Root Vegetables (Beetroot, Turnip, Carrots, Squash), Eggs, Shellfish
Zinc	Oysters, Herring, Sardines, Tuna, Shellfish Beans and Peas, Ginger, Nuts (Pecans, Almonds, Hazelnuts), Whole Grains (Wheat, Rye, Oats) Chicken, Liver, Lamb, Thyme, Cinnamon, Chilli, Mustard
Iron (Haem) (Non-Haem)	Red Meat, Chicken, Liver, Shellfish Seaweed (Kelp) Seeds (Pumpkin, Sunflower, Sesame) Nuts (Pine, Almonds, Brazil, Cashews, Walnuts, Pecan) Prunes and Prune Juice Beans (Soybean), Lentils
Chromium	Cereals (Wheat, Rye,) Root Vegetables (Carrots, Potatoes, Parsnips) Apples, Bananas, Oranges, Blueberries Pepper, Spinach
Selenium	Nuts (Brazil, Hazelnut) Cereals (Wheat, Oats, Bran, Barley) Shellfish, Root Vegetables (Turnips, Carrots, Onions) Eggs, Garlic Brown Rice
Boron	Nuts (Almonds, Hazelnuts) Fruit (Pears, Apples, Prunes) Raisins

Manganese	Liver Nuts (Pecans, Brazil, Almonds, Cashews, Walnuts) Beans Cereals (Wheat, Barley, Rye, Oats, Brown Rice) Leafy Green Vegetables, Spinach, Brussels Sprouts Beetroots, Carrots, Turnips Rhubarb Citrus Fruit Raisins
Boron	Nuts (Almonds, Hazelnuts) Fruit (Pears, Apples, Prunes) Raisins
Iodine	Seafoods including Fish, Shellfish and Seaweed Spinach Garlic Turnips Iodised salt
Silicon	Wholegrain Cereals (Barley, Oats, Brown Rice) Root Vegetables (Turnips, Parsnips, Onions, Beets) Alfalfa Seaweed Nuts (Almonds) Apples, Strawberries, Grapes
Sulphur	Root Vegetables (Onion, Turnip, Horseradish, Radish) Broccoli, Cauliflower, Cabbage Nuts Celery Watercress
Potassium	Vegetables (Potato, Carrot, Spinach, Asparagus, Tomato) Fruit (Bananas, Apricot, Avocado, Plum, Peach, Orange) Nuts (Almonds, Pecans, Cashews) Beans (Lima) Seeds (Sunflower)

7

Understanding Food Intolerances

Up to this point, we have taken a general approach to healthy eating, establishing what foods are healthy, and in what quantities. However, we now need to consider individual differences between people in order to fine-tune **YOUR** Healthy Eating Plan.

In our modern-day society, intolerances to different foods, healthy or otherwise (let alone preservatives and other man-made fillers) are all too common. **In our practice, more than 90 per cent of individuals suffer with symptoms related to such intolerances.** As the digestive system is our primary source of nourishment and detoxification, it is the first step in the journey towards physical and mental health. Even if a patient presents with problems of hormonal imbalances, for example, they will simply not be able to absorb any nutrients or herbs prescribed for their primary condition, if their digestive system is not functioning at its optimum capacity.

As Hippocrates said, 'Let food be thy medicine'. This may have been completely true in days of old; however, in the 21st century we need to discover which foods actually are medicines and which are, indeed, toxins. Once again, we need to highlight the significance of individual variances. A food for one may in fact be poison for another. Following on from this very important point is the fact that no one diet exactly suits all. There are certainly trends within specific groups, such as cultural, family and blood types. However, this truly is an oversimplification ... for, as with the rest of life, we are undoubtedly all individuals.

The reality is, any food, healthy or otherwise, may provoke a personal intolerance depending upon your own individual digestive capabilities. Commercial food processing does make food intolerances more likely, and so it is not surprising that intolerances to wheat, dairy, refined sugar foods and artificial food additives are the most likely food intolerances. However, it is simply not true that if a food is natural and considered good for you, then you are not able to develop an intolerance to it.

Take, for example, beef, apples, eggs, tomatoes, nuts and soy along with the most common food intolerances, wheat and dairy. These are surprisingly common food intolerances, despite their generally health enhancing effects in the diet of a non-intolerant person.

Interestingly, you can be:

- Intolerant to a type of food, but not to what would be considered a closely associated food. You may be intolerant to cow's milk but not goat's milk, for example.
- Intolerant to food components present across food groups, such that you display an interesting array of intolerances. For instance, an intolerance to the protein tyramine may lead to adverse reactions to foods as diverse as (but not limited to) beer and wine, cheeses, red meat and sausage, several varieties of fruit, soy sauce and sauerkraut.
- Partially tolerant to a food as long as you do not consume it in excess. For instance, you may cope with an egg every few days, but not more than this.
- Able to consume a food if raw or cooked in a particular way, but not in others. We have found people intolerant to raw apples, but not cooked apples, for example.
- Intolerant to the foods you most enjoy and/or crave. Although this may at first appear contradictory, it is explained by the body becoming addicted to hormones such as adrenaline (not unlike extreme sport junkies), that are secreted in response to the stress of consuming a food you are intolerant to, another reason why food cravings can be misleading. Some incorrectly digested foods, in particular casein (dairy) and gluten (wheat), have opioid like effects in our brains which further stimulate cravings.
- Intolerant to a food at present, but not in six months' time. Food intolerances are dynamic. They may affect you now, but if you change your ways, they may diminish or even disappear ... as

long as you keep healthy. This is why we should not follow long-term restricted diets, but regularly reassess whether or not we need to continually restrict foods that we have temporarily eliminated.

So then, do YOU have a food intolerance?

Let's ask a few simple questions. Do you experience any of the following?

1) Abdominal bloating/feeling of fullness
2) Abdominal cramps or discomfort
3) Constipation
4) Diarrhoea
5) Excess burping
6) Excess flatulence
7) Indigestion.

If you experience any one or more of these symptoms, then it is highly likely that you have one or more food intolerances, remembering that 'common things occur commonly', an important phrase that all doctors have drummed into their heads from medical school.

There are, of course, several exceptions to the rule and this is where disclaimers unfortunately apply. It is absolutely essential that you seek the opinion of a professional if your bowel habit has altered recently, if there is any blood or mucus in your stools or if you are concerned for any other reason. Sometimes food intolerances mask other sinister pathology so this point really does need to be stressed. If recurrent diarrhoea is your problem, it is also recommended that stool cultures (times three!) be sent to pathology to exclude a possible infection.

Another point to mention here is that food intolerances can be responsible for a whole range of general body symptoms. This can be understood by realising that when a food is poorly tolerated, it may also mean that it has been poorly digested by the body. This leads to the potential for large food particles to leak through the gut wall and into the blood stream. As these maldigested food chains travel around the body, they can be involved in a whole plethora of functional and organic irritations, from migraines to excess phlegm, joint pain to ear problems, vagueness and lethargy to hyperactivity. It is also possible, although uncommon, that a person experiences non-gastrointestinal symptoms due to food intolerances, without any associated gastrointestinal symptoms. Obviously you and your doctor need to exclude more serious pathology before jumping to the conclusion of food intolerance, but since a Food Elimination Regime is an easy self administered test, there is little harm in such an investigation. So, back to the task at hand.

The first step in this exercise, strangely enough, is not to change your diet at all. Rather, it is to give yourself a two-week trial of taking the maximum dose of a good probiotic (more about these in future chapters) 15 minutes before breakfast. The results are easy to interpret.

(1) If you find that 100 per cent of your original symptoms are gone, then you in fact were simply suffering from a lack of good gut bacteria (probiotics) in your diet. This is easy to remedy. We would recommend you take a full course (two-three months) of probiotics, then undertake a trial period without probiotics, or perhaps at a reduced dose. Like so many other essential 'nutrients', your body will tell you what you need to do next. If your symptoms return, then obviously you need to keep going. Simple, isn't it?

(2) If you find that some of your symptoms reduce but not all, then you are experiencing both a lack of probiotics and possible food intolerances. We recommend trialling the Food Elimination Regime that follows.

(3) If you find that you have no changes with probiotics, then it is highly probable that all your symptoms are related to food intolerances, assuming more serious pathology has been excluded.

There are, of course, other possibilities such as Candidal infections and the malabsorption of particular sugars such as fructose. Systemic Candidal infections are a point of contention amongst the medical profession. There is a conventional blood test for Candida; however, the results are controversial and must be interpreted in the light of clinical findings. The test was designed for detecting genital thrush infections in women; however, we have seen highly positive results in men with no genital infections, but all of the above symptoms (more on this in later chapters). The body's inability to properly absorb and break down certain sugars such as fructose can unfortunately at this time only be determined by specialised laboratories.

Before following the Food Elimination Regime, several other points need to be clarified. Food intolerances are not food allergies. They involve different immune system components (IgG compared with IgE) and being tested for allergies does not automatically mean that you have been tested for intolerances. Food intolerances will not kill you like severe food allergies that lead to anaphylaxis, but they can insidiously creep into your life and slowly eat away at your energy, your wellbeing and your happiness.

After you perform the Food Elimination Regime, you will discover so much about your body's own intelligence. Furthermore, the Food Elimination Regime is an effective body detoxification, resulting for the majority of individuals in significant weight loss.

So if you are looking for that all important 'kick-start' to your diet, here it is in a form that will not only shed the kilos, but also educate you to your body's own personal food intolerances.

In the end it is not up to us or another health professional to tell you what you can and cannot eat. Like many other journeys in life, it is impossible to ignore the wisdom inherent within, once you have been enlightened. And no, that does not mean we should all be puritans on restricted diets, but rather that we should make our own informed choices. We would simply not be human if we chose not to eat the beautiful food at that gala night out (or the wine) to save ourselves some excess flatulence the following day!

As the saying goes, 'Everything in moderation'. However, you must accept the consequences of any decision you make. If you do choose to continually eat foods that are toxic to your body, then you will increase your intestinal permeability (leaky gut), which will then cause you to experience greater sensitivity to your environment and further food intolerances. Remember, the choice is yours. But more importantly, remember you do actually have a choice. More often than not, this is forgotten in the chaos of life.

8

The Food Elimination Regime

To establish whether or not you are intolerant to a food, you should participate in an Elimination Diet. You will need to follow this diet plan carefully, realising that all aspects of the plan, including both food elimination AND reintroduction, are essential to the process.

Although intended primarily to determine the presence of Food Intolerances, the Food Elimination program also serves as both a detoxication and an advanced weight loss program (a 'kick-start').

Establishing foods to be eliminated from your diet

Food intolerances are individual, and different people will be intolerant to different foods. Therefore the choice of foods to be eliminated from your diet needs to be individually established according to your own personal constitution. The foods to be eliminated will be established according to:

1. The most frequently experienced food intolerances experienced by the general population (common things occur commonly).
2. Food intolerances most commonly associated with your medical history.
3. Foods that you crave or are addicted to (like the alcoholic, many people crave foods that are both addictive and detrimental to their health due to an addiction to the adrenaline secreted when the body is stressed).

Foods That You Are Allowed Include

- All vegetables
- Most fruits other than apples, oranges, strawberries, pineapples and tomatoes
- All meats other than beef (such as pork, chicken, fish, lamb)
- Rice and rice products (such as rice pasta and rice syrup for sweetening).

Foods That You Are NOT Allowed Include

- **WHEAT, YEAST AND GLUTEN**

    Avoid all wheat-based products including breads, pastas, couscous biscuits etc

    Check labels carefully for gluten and wheat, particularly in sauces (e.g. soy sauces)

    Exclude all yeast products such as breads, cookies, cakes, Vegemite, Marmite and many salad dressings and soups (check food labels)

- **OATS AND RYE**
- **DAIRY**

    Exclude all types of dairy products such as cheese, yoghurt etc made from cow's milk.

    Avoid products with casein, whey and lactose on the food labels

- **BEEF AND PRESERVED MEATS**
- **PEANUTS, PEANUT BUTTER, PEANUT OIL, SESAME**
- **SOY PRODUCTS** (if you include these within your usual diet)

    Exclude soy milk, tofu, tempeh, soy sauce and other food derivatives. Check labels for soy products

- ✦ EGGS AND EGG PRODUCTS
- ✦ ORANGES
- ✦ TOMATOES
- ✦ STRAWBERRIES, PINEAPPLES, APPLE
- ✦ CHOCOLATE PRODUCTS
- ✦ ALL PROCESSED FOODS AND ADDED SUGARS
- ✦ FOOD ADDITIVES AND PRESERVATIVES

    — Therefore exclude most packaged products and all confectionaries

- ✦ COFFEE, TEA, SOFT DRINKS, FRUIT JUICES
- ✦ ALCOHOL
- ✦ TAP WATER

This is by no means an exhaustive list, but it does include most of the foods that individuals are most frequently intolerant to.

YOU SHOULD ADD ANY FOOD YOU PERSONALLY SUSPECT MAY CAUSE YOU ANY SYMPTOMS OF FOOD INTOLERANCE (SEE LIST THAT FOLLOWS). FURTHERMORE, YOU MAY ALSO CONSIDER ANY FOOD YOU COMPULSIVELY EAT TO ESTABLISH IF YOUR CONSUMPTION IS DUE TO PREFERENCE OR ADDICTION.

SIMPLIFIED MEAL PLAN: 3 WEEKS

After identifying the foods to be eliminated from your diet you will now follow a simplified meal plan for the following **three weeks**. As you are on a restricted diet, you might consider the use of supplemental meals in the form of protein powders, but you must obviously check the ingredients of these for eliminated foods as well. For the Elimination Diet to be successful you must be committed 100 per cent to the simplified diet, especially if you are eliminating foods to which you have cravings.

Breakfast

Examples include non-wheat-based cereals available commercially or homemade muesli (no oats) from wholefood stores. Allowed fruits can be added. Rice milk, nut milk or non-cow's milk yoghurt may also be used. Consider using unsweetened fruit juice from bottled pears, peaches, apricots and plums over your cereal instead of a milk substitute. Alternatively, a fruit smoothie or grilled vegetables with lamb/fish.

Lunch

Examples include unlimited amounts of salad (excluding tomatoes) and vegetables—any type of meat or fish, other than beef. Try avocado, pine nuts, feta cheese (non-cow's milk). Olive oil, lemon juice and fresh herbs for dressings. Don't forget dinner leftovers with rice/corn cakes. Sushi with tamari (for those not eliminating soy) is also an excellent option. (NB: wasabi contains lactose and is not therefore allowed).

Dinner

Examples include all vegetables, salad, chicken, fish, lamb, veal, pork, chickpeas, lentils and other legumes. Rice, rice vermicelli and bean sprout vermicelli can also be used. Grated carrots and zucchini can be used to replace pasta. Check your local health food store for many new wheat and dairy substitutes.

Snacks

Examples include nuts (not peanuts), most fruits, seeds, fresh vegetables, acceptable dips, fruit smoothies, herbal teas and filtered water.

Please note that quite frequently people will initially feel worse on the diet, despite the diet being based on fresh or simply cooked meals. This usually occurs as the body withdraws from foods that it craves, not unlike withdrawal from other addictions. Symptoms may include headaches, nausea, dizziness, gastrointestinal upset, fatigue, poor concentration, lethargy and irritability. Coffee withdrawals, in particular, often mean headaches.

You must therefore make sure you drink at least six–eight cups of water during your simplified diet to reduce these effects. This period should usually pass in three–four days.

FOOD CHALLENGE PROCESS: 3–4 WEEKS

This is the most important aspect of the Elimination Diet, but also the most often incorrectly performed. This is because many people feel better after being on an Elimination Diet and therefore choose to remain on the limited food plan, ignoring the Food Challenge stage. In doing this, they risk continuing to exclude many foods they are not intolerant to, because they have not been specific enough in identifying their own individual triggers. Not only will this deny a person the pleasure of eating a wide variety of foods, it will also risk future nutritional deficiencies.

Food Challenges are performed by reintroducing each eliminated food one at a time every three days. You may reintroduce your foods in whatever order you choose. However, it is preferable to re-introduce dairy, wheat and refined sugars last as your detoxification time will be longer.

It is important that you introduce each food component separately. For example, introduce pasta when introducing wheat. Then you may try different types of bread—yeast-free, gluten-free, rye, spelt, usual wheat-containing bread. If complex foods such as a chocolate muffin are used for re-introduction first, it will be impossible to determine which component of the food is responsible for a reaction.

For example, on Day 1 of your reintroduction phase, you introduce eggs. Eat one egg and note if any reactions occur. If not, then the next day, eat two or three eggs. Challenge your body and again note any responses. If there are not any responses, keep eggs in your diet and the next day introduce another food. However, if you do get a reaction to a particular food, then you must remove that food from your diet as it will interfere with the responses from other foods you are yet to introduce. Also, wait until the symptoms dissipate before you introduce your next food.

You should keep a record of your signs and symptoms during your food re-introduction. This will allow you to more accurately establish which foods are causing your symptoms.

The following are symptoms you should be aware of, and therefore should note in your diary:

- The most common symptoms are those related to the gastro-intestinal tract itself including:
  - Nausea
  - Bloating
  - Vomiting
  - Diarrhoea
  - Constipation
  - Flatulence
  - Heartburn
  - Abdominal pain

- Fatigue, light-headedness, vagueness
- Hyperactivity and irritability
- Difficulty concentrating, emotional instability
- Migraine and headaches
- Aching or swollen joints
- Muscle aches
- Wheezes, coughs, sinusitis or phlegm
- Sore throat, bad taste in mouth
- Dark bags or circles under eyes
- Skin rashes
- Genital itch or vaginitis.

OR ANY OTHER SIGN OR SYMPTOM THAT HAS LESSENED OR DISAPPEARED DURING THE FOOD ELIMINATION PHASE THAT REOCCURS WITH THE REINTRODUCTION OF SPECIFIC FOODS.

Certain individuals may be intolerant to food components that cross food groups such as salicylates, amines and fructose. The following gives examples of foods from each of these groups. It is strongly advisable to seek professional help if you feel you may have these particular intolerances as such restricted diets may result in major nutritional deficiencies.

Salicylates
Apricots, asparagus, beetroot, capsicum, carrot, corn, cranberry, cucumber, dried fruit, herbs, onions, mango, peppermint, plum, prune, pumpkin, raspberry (and other berries), rockmelon, spices, sultanas, sweet potato, watermelon, zucchini.

Fructose
Apples, Pears, Peaches, Oranges, Prunes, Raisins, Tropical Fruits, Figs, Juices of same, Corn Syrup (soft drinks, canned foods) or too much of fruit in total in a short period.

Amines
Intolerances to a series of proteins including histamine, tyramine and phenylalanine. Chocolate, cheese, wine, beer, salted fish, broad beans, avocado, banana, raspberry, pawpaw.

Nightshades
Tomatoes, eggplants, capsicum, chillies.

Oxalates
Nuts, spinach, berries, figs, rhubarb, wholewheat bread, oatmeal, sesame and sunflower seeds, soy, chocolates, beets, celery, eggplants, green beans, leeks, many herbs, green capsicum, rhubarb, squash, turnip.

Food Additives and Preservatives
Often implicated in food intolerances, a range of food additives and preservatives can cause a variety of symptoms on a person by person basis. However the list of additive numbers that may cause problems is long, so you will need to put on your detective hat if you are not to overly restrict your diet. Common additives to consider include the Metabisulphite group (220–224—many dried fruits), Nitrites and nitrates (249–251—processed deli-meats), MSG (restaurant foods, soups and sauces) and colours (another long list, look at the colour of the food instead).

FINAL DIET

Once you are aware of what foods you are intolerant to, you will be able to modify your diet. It is important to make your diet as varied in food intake as possible within the limitations of the foods that you have discovered affect you. Try and look for alternative sources of vitamin and minerals which you may otherwise lose from your diet due to the loss of key foods (see tables in Section 4, Chapter 2).

Finally, there are several key points to reiterate about food intolerances that affect your choice of diet in the long term.

- Unlike classic food allergies, food intolerances are dynamic in nature. This means that being intolerant to a food today does not mean you will be intolerant in the future.
- Doctor or practitioner led programs aiming to improve the function of the gastrointestinal tract often help to minimise the effects of established food intolerances. The more committed you are to such programs, the more likely your success in overcoming a food intolerance.
- Food intolerances are often determined by the quantity of food you consume. Small amounts of foods that you are sensitive to may be tolerated, especially if other health factors have been maximised. However, the boundaries between tolerance and sensitivity must be carefully established if you choose to consume foods that you have previously reacted to.
- Healthy eating patterns, reduction in stress, reduced alcohol intake, reductions in certain medications and other health enhancing factors will maximise your potential for overcoming a food intolerance.

It therefore pays to intermittently reassess your food intolerances with occasional challenges just to make sure that you cannot re-introduce foods you might previously have reacted to.

Remember to take care for unless you show balance and restraint, you may risk returning to the overindulgences and cravings of the past.

IMPORTANT NOTE:

Food Allergies with risk of Anaphylaxis: Anaphylaxis is an abnormal or exaggerated immune system response to specific food proteins, that may lead to symptoms of facial and/ or airways swelling, cardiovascular shutdown, skin reactions, abdominal pain, and, in a small number, even death. Foods most commonly indicated include peanuts, milk, eggs, tree nuts, soy and fish, although many other foods have also been implicated in individual cases (wheat, banana, kiwi fruit, mustard and food preservatives) whether eaten, touched or smelt.

CARE OF THIS CONDITION SHOULD BE UNDER THE SUPERVISION OF A MEDICAL SPECIALIST DUE TO THE SMALL BUT PRESENT RISK OF ANAPHYLAXIS AND DEATH.

9

Eat Out and Enjoy

Here is a simple question to ask yourself. Is your local fast food surprise good for you? Use common sense here. Don't fall for the advertising. Most likely not. Is it going to kill you to eat at a fast food store one or two times per week? No, contrary to the health obsessed gurus, probably not.

What about a quality restaurant? Is the menu necessarily balanced? No. Full of creamy riches and dreamy pastries? Yes. Overladen with carbohydrates or mass protein servings? Possibly. Is eating one or two meals a week in such a restaurant going to kill you? No. It probably won't even harm you. After all, your body has detoxification systems for a reason!

Puritans be damned, good food is a celebration of life as much as it is a nutrient! So a vital lesson in keeping to a simple healthy diet is this: 90 per cent is good enough. And good enough means no self-blame. Enjoy. Guilt, as in most areas of life, is a useless emotion when it comes to food.

What if you are eating more than three meals a week at a restaurant of whatever quality?

If you do this, you are going to have to make a few choices. The most obvious one is stop doing it. Start to eat in a healthier manner by taking time to prepare meals at home. If this is your choice, the healthy eating rules are simple. You already know them.

But this is not the only solution. You might also continue to eat out but make healthier restaurant choices.

If so, your answer is to request meals that follow the healthy eating guidelines. First of all remember, you have the choice. It is your dollar a restaurant wants, so you get to ask for a little individual consideration. Be assertive. Once a restaurant knows you will come back they are more often than not going to accommodate your wishes.

Another choice you have is whether or not to eat or leave what is on your plate. Make the choice to leave foods that are served in excess or out of balance to your needs. This includes bread. Remember, you can eat an open sandwich with a knife and fork, you don't need to eat both slices provided. Nor do you need to eat the chips or potatoes, or lap up the remaining sauce, however good it tastes.

Otherwise here are a few simple guidelines for making eating out healthy. Remember, they only need apply if you are eating out more than two to three meals a week. Less than this and enjoy what you want, no questions asked.

- Avoid **fast food restaurants and bakeries**. Save your money and spend it on one or two meals a week at a decent quality restaurant. Remember too that most 'healthy food choices' in corner stores or food courts still depend upon sandwich buns or pre-cut salads that become devoid of nutrients if left too long.
- Look for **sandwich or salad bars** that are prepared to cut and, where necessary, cook your meals as you wait, rather than pre-cut and display. The same rule applies for most buffet style meals. If the food is ready to serve and you don't know how long it has been on display, don't eat it.
- When eating **Australian pub or American ranch style** meals, 'meat and three veg' is a reasonable option, given one vegetable will be a potato. Either this or choose a side salad. You could also try trading your inevitable chips, fries or fried wedges for an extra serving of vegetables or salad. It is likely that your meat cut will be high fat for taste unless otherwise specified (remove this) and overly large (you don't need to eat the whole half kilogram slab!). Sausages are most often high in fat content as well. These, along with fried 'English' style breakfasts, should be avoided in preference to a more 'Continental' style breakfast including muesli (oat based is preferable) and fruit (but not the pastry).
- Eating **Italian**? Remember that modern Italian food has had its dimensions twisted. Pastas come super-sized, pizzas thick crusted and pan-fried and cheese oozes over the lot. The Mediterranean miracle lives in Italy, but not in many Italian restaurants elsewhere. Downsize your pizza or pasta to an entrée serving (½ cup cooked

pasta or 1–2 slices pizza only), and look for a main of lean meat, roasted chicken or seafood with an exquisite salad and olive oil based herb infused salad dressing or roast vegetable platter.

✦ Eating **French or Continental**? The desserts, the pastries, the rich sauces and fried delights … well, how often do you eat French? This said, you're better off with grilled and baked mains or seafood and fresh fruit desserts. Otherwise be careful with the additional carbohydrate servings.

✦ When eating **Spanish** food, do not overdo the rice in paella and other such dishes, whilst tapas provides you with the wonderful opportunity to indulge in many different flavours … just be careful about how much bread you take in dripping up the lavish sauces. But again, how often do you eat Spanish?

✦ When eating at **Chinese, Thai, Vietnamese** or **Indonesian** restaurants, avoid deep-fried foods including fried rice and entrees such as spring rolls. Instead choose steamed or stir-fried meals or clear soups. Beware of rich sauces. You may have to search for vegetables in many Chinese meals with the exception of onions, baby corn and the occasional floret of broccoli, despite the opposite being the case in a peasant village in China! Ask for a side serve of steamed vegetables where this is the case otherwise you are likely to fill yourself up with protein, sauce and rice.

✦ Eating **Japanese**? Sushi and sashimi are excellent raw foods, and miso a healthy soup. Otherwise the same rules apply as for other Asian cuisine. Tempura, being deep-fried, is not the best option.

✦ Your biggest risk when eating **Indian** is filling up on rice and naan bread, followed by the delightful sauces your meat and vegetables will be blended with. Go instead for curries, which are a healthier option and likely to satisfy you faster than most other foods, particularly if you are drinking lots of cool water with them. Limit your intake of deep-fried foods such as samosas and bhaji. Yes, there is often dairy in Indian foods, but it is both heated and sourced from yoghurt, aiding digestion. Ensure you delight in the vast array or herbs and spices found in every recipe, an important premise of traditional Ayurvedic medicine.

- When eating **Mexican**, it's just too easy to overeat corn chips and then to follow up with a taco, burrito, fajitas or other high carbohydrate wrap. But Mexican can provide a very healthy balance of meat, rice, beans and vegetables if the former are overlooked or consumed in moderation. Salsa and guacamole (within reason) are healthy when used as condiments.
- Eating **Middle Eastern** cuisine? Careful with the quality of the meat on the rotisserie, it is often high in fat.

And if you are eating Zimbabwean, Bolivian or Icelandic cuisine? Well how often do you eat it unless you live in Africa, Bolivia or Iceland? (in which case the general healthy eating rules apply). So make it one of your celebration meals in the week and love it!

Is the point of this chapter clear yet? It should be. Enjoy up to two–three unrestricted meals per week (whether at home or in restaurants). After which focus on balancing your eating plan as well as you can and without excuse.

In other words, when you indulge, do it well, enjoy.
Love your food, love the taste, love your life.
Because 90 per cent right is all right if you keep it simple.
And then the other 10 per cent can be as sexy as you like!

10

Drink and Be Merry

Let's make a toast, to a short and simple chapter! If you have ears, you know the truth of it. Excess alcohol is not good for your health, your wealth, your relationships, your life, or the morning after. No new news here!

Nor will it probably come as any surprise that two standard drinks of alcohol per day may have health benefits. Such moderate consumption might be cardioprotective, improve circulation, dementia and may even provide some protection against the risk of Diabetes Mellitus (Type 2). On the down side, there may be an increase in the risk of some cancers at this level of consumption, although the evidence is not clear-cut.

- ✦ But these comments apply to one to two standard drinks of alcohol per day, not drinking yourself silly. So as it stands now, enjoy your two standard drinks per day.
- ✦ How much alcohol in a standard drink? Here is where you will need to read the label. Why? Because a standard drink is measured by alcohol content, which varies between different drinks, even if of the same type. Every alcohol label is required to show the standard drink size due to drink driving laws, so this should not be hard to find.
- ✦ What about coffee? On the downside, coffee is an adrenal stimulant, which is why you like it when you need energy or are stressed. It also affects absorption of certain minerals (iron and zinc amongst them), and may affect blood pressure. On the upside, it may help control blood sugar rises and decrease the risk of dementia.

So yet again, health seems to be about balance. As long as you consume coffee in moderation and don't make it a substitute for breakfast, or any other meal. A good guide is generally one to two **REAL** coffees daily with the occasional cappuccino when out. Your body and mind will generally tell you how much you can tolerate. If you experienced headaches during the withdrawal stage of your Food Elimination Regime, it is highly likely that you were drinking too much coffee.

As for tea, generally one to two cups a day is not a problem. Try different herbal teas, or green teas, with lemon and lime. Make your own by boiling pineapple skins in a saucepan of water.

Coffee and tea have diuretic effects, so don't solely include them in your quest for fluids (If you are following the healthy eating approach in this book fluid intake should not be a problem, as you will be getting plenty of fluids from your food, as well as the additional fluid intake we are recommending.)

So a final joyous word. If you are going to drink alcohol, but in moderation, go for quality. Same with coffee; get a grinder and explore all the delicious bean flavours (or if you don't drink coffee, just the aromas!) As for teas, try a whole variety of herbal delights as well as mainstream flavours.

Let's face it. Life is going to kill you in the end, however well you live it. So enjoy a little quality, and don't look back!

11

So What About Your Weight?

Are you asking yourself this question?

Healthy eating sounds great, but I want to look trim.

Don't panic. If you follow this diet you will certainly lose weight but only as is appropriate to your own individual constitution.

If you followed our advice and performed the Food Elimination Regime, then it is highly likely that you have already shed some extra kilograms, are feeling better within yourself, experiencing more energy and motivation and are wiser to your body's wisdom as to which foods are healthy and not healthy **FOR YOU**.

Be careful if you are someone who feels so much better and/or has lost weight on the Food Elimination Regime to the point where you haven't re-introduced excluded foods.

If this is the case, go back and read the chapter on the Food Elimination Regime. You must perform the reintroduction phase. Reintroduction is indeed the most important part of the regime, as it will give you the knowledge you require for long-term healthy living.

Don't be concerned that you will lose the benefits of the regime in doing this. The Healthy Eating Plan will keep you moving forward in a more controlled and healthy fashion. And besides, you now should know the foods that were most likely to have been causing you discomfort and weight gain, and should have removed them from your personalised Healthy Eating Plan.

As for the long-term, weight loss of no more than one half kilogram per week should be the maximum you aim for after the initial gains in the first two weeks (which can be reasonably impressive due to fluid loss, up to four kilograms or more). Any more than this is risky dieting, with a high chance of weight rebound or other more serious complications in the future.

What about nutritional supplementation?

If you want to try nutritional supplementation see Section 5, Chapter 6, 'Insulin Resistance, Diabetes and Weight Loss', and the forewords to other relevant chapters. The supplements you choose to aid weight loss will depend on your individual health state and the reason why you have put on weight in the first place. There are various reasons, both proven and theorised, as to why people put on weight, but establishing which is most pertinent to you is the difficulty. For this reason suggesting a generalised supplement program for weight loss is, at best, a guess. You really do need to personalise your approach to get additional results from supplementation above and beyond the gains made through diet and exercise alone.

Which brings us to an appropriate place for a reminder:

Don't forget exercise! For any diet without exercise is, at best, a half measure.

What if I'm still not losing weight?

If after trying not just this eating approach, but many others, and despite committing yourself to an exercise program and doing everything suggested, you still have not lost weight, then it's time to look at medical reasons for your weight gain or inability to lose weight.

Please note that we are not including those who have lost weight, then put it back on. If this is the case you know how to lose it again, after which you need to commit to stabilising yourself on the Healthy Eating Plan. No, we mean if you have absolutely not lost weight on this or any other diet plan at the rate suggested above over the long-term.

This means it's time to consult a medical practitioner who can carry out appropriate tests to establish the cause of your inability to lose weight while eating healthily. Generally there are three main medical reasons why this may be the case: insulin resistance, oestrogen dominance and hypothyroidism. We suggest you start by looking at relevant chapters in section 5, but emphasise that pathology tests are required here to guide you.

12

The Recipe-less Recipe Guide

Most books about diets come with a long list of recipes, often with unusual or expensive ingredients. It is more than likely you have several in your kitchen bookshelf right now. Meanwhile, you are certain to have a number of other recipe books ready for you to explore, filled with a mix of tempting and variably healthy suggestions.

So do you need another recipe book to get you through the next two, six or 12 week period of power-packed health change you have planned?

Or do you have to learn a new way of cooking?

Or combining foods?

Not at all, for you already have 1001 recipes at your disposal.

90 per cent of meals, assuming they involve the healthy cooking methods outlined in the text (Salads, Soups, Steaming, Stir-Frying, Grilling, Roasting, Casseroles) will be usable if you only take a moment of preparation time to consider how they fit into your Healthy Eating Plan. And the other 10 per cent (or those involving less healthy foods or methods of cooking) you can use for your meals or days left to beautiful guilt-free sinful delight.

All that's needed are a few simple changes to most home cooked whole food recipes.

Photocopy the following guide with the Serving Size Guide (pages 96–97) and Variety of the Main Plate Chart (page 99) and place on your kitchen wall, reviewing them every time you wish to try a new or rejuvenated recipe, and you will go forward on your Healthy Eating Plan.

A Guide to Modifying Recipes

1. Identify any personal Food Intolerances in the recipe and limit or find an alternative food to provide a similar flavour. This will be the major determinant of whether or not you can follow a recipe.
2. Adapt the number and size of cereal/grain and/or starch vegetable serves (potato, sweet potato, corn) you have had and plan to have in your day. Consult serving size tables when you dish out. Get this right. Do not overeat from the cereal/grain or starch vegetable group. This is all too common since this group often forms the base to the rest of your foods, being put on the plate first to absorb the flavours of the rest of the meal.
3. Adapt recipes where possible for the amount of dairy you will consume in your day (1 cup total).

THE ABOVE THREE GUIDELINES WILL PREDOMINANTLY DETERMINE WHETHER OR NOT YOU ARE ABLE TO ADAPT A RECIPE FOR HEALTHY EATING, ASSUMING YOU HAVE CHOSEN A HEALTHY COOKING STYLE AS OUTLINED IN THE TEXT.

4. Estimate your red meat, poultry or fish serve by the hand method. This commonly used measure estimates a red meat serving as the thickness and length of your palm (remove fat), poultry as a palm and half finger length (remove skin) and seafood as a full hand length.
5. Add the legume/pulses group as you choose, preferably at least ½ to 1 cup per day.
6. Fill your plate with as many vegetables as you like so that you feel satisfied with your main meal.
7. Adding whole fruits as desired, with the noted limitations on tropical and dried fruits of one serve only at any one sitting.
8. Predominantly flavour your meals with fresh or dried herbs, vinegar, yoghurt, lemon juice or olive oil. Add fresh herbs after cooking to retain flavour.
9. Use dressing and sauces sparingly as a light coat to your foods rather than poured on. If you do this you will not need to limit

their use. On the other hand, if you frequently swim your food through sauces, you may need to limit how often you make them and restrict them to your pleasure meals.

10. Consume a glass of water with your meal before any other fluid (6–8 glasses of water per day).
11. Consume levels of alcohol, coffee, tea and fruit juices at any meal as appropriate to your day's total serves (one–two serves).
12. And once the food is on the plate, do not assume you need to eat it all. If you feel content (rather than a bloated 'full'), stop eating. If, as is normal, your rice, pasta, potato etc has been placed on your plate first in order to soak up the sauces or juices of the meal, they should also be the food group left on the plate if you have over-served.

SECTION 4

Examining the Health and Treatment Continuum

Life is a continuum from wellness to illness and an integrated approach to medical care should ideally reflect this. In health we address optimal wellness through lifestyle modification, exercise and diet but, while these remain pertinent throughout our whole health experience, we may reach a point where stronger interventions are more appropriate.

The key to optimal health in the presence of disease is a minimalist approach to treatment, while still achieving results.

Where we can achieve a result through simple healthy living rather than nutritional supplementation, this should be our path. Where effective nutritional supplementation is preferable to prescription medication use due to minimal risk of side effects, this should be chosen. Yet ultimately, when organ decline or failure are present, or discomfort reaches the point where nutritional (or other natural health) interventions are not working, conventional medical approaches may be necessary, be they prescriptive medication, surgery, chemotherapy, radiotherapy or otherwise.

Yet a truly integrated approach to medical care is not a step by step path through the different levels of therapy. It is a mutually co-operative integration of lifestyle modification, nutritional supplementation and other complementary approaches with medication prescription and surgery as necessary.

We must ramp up the power of our interventions as required to treat acute phases of dysfunction and disease, after which we then wean back our care to a level at which the Mindbody can re-establish its own self-directed health maintenance to the best of its ability.

1

Health, Dysfunction, Disease: When Should You Intervene?

We would all like to have Optimal Health. However, many people will come to this book in a less than optimal condition. Perhaps you have been diagnosed with a disease—cardiac disease, diabetes, inflammatory bowel disease. Or maybe you have a series of non-specific health concerns that have not been diagnosed or which you do not consider important enough to tell your doctor. Such symptoms often include excess flatulence, abdominal bloating, alternating diarrhoea and constipation, inconsistent muscle aches and pains, excess sleepiness, poor clarity of thoughts and mood swings, for example.

Either way, one or more of your body systems is likely to be in a state of dysfunction. Through accumulated neglect or the bad luck of your genetic predisposition, your body is not working optimally and you are experiencing the consequences. Indeed, any sign or symptom from your body should be considered carefully. Less than optimal health does not arise while your body is working correctly. All negative signs and symptoms indicate some sort of mind and/or body dysfunction, whether you, your doctor or anybody else knows exactly what it is or not.

So what is dysfunction?

Dysfunction is when a cell, organ or system is not working how it should be. The job is simply not being done properly; information is not being interpreted correctly, building blocks are not being constructed according to specification, toxins, micro-organisms and mutant cells are not being eradicated from the body.

And why are our cells, organs and systems not functioning correctly?

While genetics may play a part, it is rarely the case that your family inheritance alone means a predetermined sentence of disease. For dysfunction to arise, you also need an accumulation of negative health influences to occur as a consequence of neglect of the healthy lifestyle principles we have discussed in the first half of this book. Unhealthy life experiences (whether through choice or misfortune), lack of exercise, smoking and poor diet are just a few of these significant risk factors for both dysfunction and disease.

Cellular, organ or system dysfunction certainly precedes cellular, organ or system disease. So when do you have a dysfunction and when do you have a disease?

In reality, the defining line is arbitrary. In truth, the line from health to dysfunction and on to disease is more often than not ill-defined, other than for a combination of dynamic investigative reports based on population averages. All too often these statistical ranges are used to decide whether or not a person has a disease, irrespective of clinical presentation. Furthermore, the clinical relevance of most tests are directed towards diagnosing disease states long after dysfunctional cell, organ or systems performance have been well established.

There are definite disease states clearly marked by critical events such as stroke or myocardial infarct (heart attack), but even in such circumstances these events are in the majority triggered by a slow decline in healthy function such as high cholesterol, leading to atherosclerosis, preceding the critical incidence of occlusion, clot formation or embolic breakaway. **We simply do not fall from a state of health on one day to wake up with diabetes the next.** Cancer cells do not grow from naught to diagnostic levels overnight. Diseases are triggered by defining events but preceded by a build up in dysfunction prior to critical decline.

But where do these disease-preceding dysfunctions find voice? Are they somehow hiding their presence, or are they in fact communicating with us despite our ignorance to the facts of the matter? The latter is most certainly the case, for our health dysfunctions do present us with symptoms in the day to day, in the physical irritations we experience. Muscle aches and pains, flatulence, bloating, diarrhoea and constipation, cramping, frequent infections, clouded thinking ('brain fog'), low fitness levels and so forth. These are the indicators of dysfunction that precede formalised disease classifications as marked by objective clinical measures.

There are warning signs for many oncoming diseases, even if we are not used to listening to and interpreting them.

Don't be alarmed. Most early warning signs aren't telling you that you are about to get a major disease tomorrow (although some, such as blood in the faeces, must be acted upon immediately). These warning signs are telling you that you have a cellular, organ or system dysfunction. These are dysfunctions that you can do something about before they develop into disease, if you so choose to intervene. In fact, it is often the case that such symptoms linger for weeks, months and even years, if we choose to ignore or accept these minor discomforts as a normal baseline of wellness. Such is the resilience of our bodies, particularly in our youth, that we can often persist in a state of dysfunction for long periods before serious consequences manifest.

Since dysfunction always precedes disease, there are as a consequence key relationships between system dysfunctions and diagnosable disease states. But further to this, single system dysfunctions can lead to multiple disease states depending upon an individual's particular susceptibility. This is the reason why many people, once given a chronic disease diagnosis, accumulate further chronic diagnoses over time, unless the underlying system or systems dysfunctions are correctly identified and subsequently treated.

This is highlighted by the recent categorisation of 'Syndrome X', a term describing a variety of disease states; obesity, insulin resistance, hyperglycaemia, high blood pressure and high cholesterol.

The medical system far too often sees simply a cluster of different diseases, and thus in turn prescribes an ever-increasing sum of prescription drugs. It would be far more sensible to treat the predisposing dysfunction, for example, Insulin Resistance, and minimise multi-drug prescription to the specific residual dysfunctions that are left unaddressed.

What we learn from such a condition is the importance of attempting to treat the underlying dysfunctions that precede disease, rather than wait for disease to reach a level of clinically defined diagnosis. For we can address

Insulin Resistance prior to it becoming diabetes, high cholesterol before it progresses into atherosclerosis and heart attack, a lack of good gut bacteria and recognition of food intolerances before it is diagnosed as irritable bowel syndrome. As long as we acknowledge the symptoms that underlie these dysfunctions, rather than ignoring them as irrelevant discomforts. Indeed few symptoms are ever irrelevant if you understand what they indicate.

Of course we are talking in the main about the more prevalent chronic diseases. Less frequent and often genetically related diseases are obscure enough to hide their sinister faces prior to our detection. Other diseases may catch us unawares because we are still unsure why they arise, particularly autoimmune disorders. Similarly cancer is an evil foe that can also go unnoticed for some time without giving us a clue to its presence. In these instances we can only hope to combat our predisposed risk by maintaining the highest level of wellbeing possible, through healthy eating, exercise, stress reduction, sleep, and the treatment of noticeable dysfunction as it arises.

So when should we treat a disorder? When it is a dysfunction or when it is a disease? Well preferably, before it ever happens. As the saying goes, 'prevention is better than cure'.

If your body doesn't reach a state of dysfunction, it will never reach a state of disease. Keep your body healthy, and this whole conversation never need happen.

But given that you have noticed irregularities in your health, however minor the symptoms, it's best to act now. For the sooner you act, the less you will need to do. And the easier it will be to do whatever is necessary.

- ✦ Act before dysfunctions arise and—unless genetically predisposed or as a consequence of a traumatic event—you will simply need to follow healthy, happy living principles to avoid disease.
- ✦ Act in the early stages of disharmony, and you may only need to choose several specific interventions to return you to a state of normality.
- ✦ Act in a state of system dysfunction and more work needs to be done, perhaps a few supplements taken, but the dysfunction can still be overcome.

EXAMINING THE HEALTH AND TREATMENT CONTINUUM

- Leave intervention until disease is diagnosed, and medications may be in order, perhaps surgery, or other drastic interventions.
- Allow disease to decline, and life becomes complicated. You may need to take multiple prescription drugs, perhaps have surgery, chemotherapy or radiotherapy, with the risk of side effects. Treatments become more complicated.
- Accumulate multiple disease states, and you really are behind the eight ball.

So if dysfunction or disease exist, when should you seek help from a health practitioner, and when can you treat your condition yourself with simple measures such as those found in this book?

This depends on how much interest you take in your own health and what you are willing to do to maintain it. Even when in seemingly good health, there is an argument for consulting health professionals for the best of advice for maintaining that health. You have a choice, therefore, to seek advice even in good health! This, in effect, is what you are doing when you ask a gym instructor for advice. Similarly, you can stretch this approach to seeing a nutritionist or doctor for personalised diet and supplement advice, or a counsellor, psychologist or life coach for mentoring.

It is in your best interests to seek advice from professionals who share this approach to health. Otherwise, your doctor or other health professional may simply try to reassure you that nothing is wrong, despite your personal discomfort, since their view of ill health begins much further down the wellness/illness paradigm than yours.

On the other hand, when **MUST** you see a health professional regarding your health concerns is, perhaps, a more important question. In particular, when should medical care be under the overall guidance of a medical doctor?

Here are few guidelines.

1. When you have multiple serious signs and symptoms for which you have no obvious answer.
2. When you require pathology testing and interpretation for your signs and symptoms.

3. When you are already undergoing complex medical procedures (e.g. chemotherapy, radiotherapy, surgical procedures).
4. When you are taking prescription medication that may interact with any change in lifestyle including diet, herb or supplement use.
5. When you have a condition that involves an irreversible disease state (post Myocardial Infarct, emphysema, renal failure).
6. For complex genetic, autoimmune, cancer or other such diseases.
7. When your overall medical condition is made complex by the involvement of two or more body systems.
8. For psychological states that you cannot control, and in particular, when you are at risk of harming yourself or others.
9. When you have been previously hospitalised for a currently active disease state that you are seeking help with.
10. When the set of signs and symptoms that concern you, however minor, are resistant to simple lifestyle change and self-administered interventions after a three–month period.

This is not to say that a medical doctor is definitely the best person to treat your condition. On the contrary, most of what follows by way of intervention for cellular, organ or systems dysfunction, and therefore, in turn, disease states, involve natural medicines which are prescribable by a naturopath, nutritionist/dietician, herbalist or similar, whether or not medical drugs are used concurrently. However, once complex pathology testing, drug prescription or medical procedures are instituted, someone must be able to ensure that co-occurring interventions do not lead to negative consequences as a result of unfavourable interactions.

Yes, your doctor needs to know what natural interventions you are deciding to follow. This is essential as soon as he or she reaches for a prescription pad. What if he or she doesn't want to know? Or tells you not to undertake self treatment despite you having thoroughly researched your chosen intervention?

Ask for their reason. Listen carefully. Is their response based on a sound medical argument (for example, risk of drug-diet, drug-nutrient or drug-herb interactions), or a personal bias against natural medicine? Be reasonable yourself in listening to their justification.

What do you do when you do not accept their answer?

Remember, you are the consumer. Seek a medical doctor who suits your needs, who will provide you with a balanced approach to your health states, and who is willing to consider the treatment of health in as proactive a manner as you, including using the assistance of whatever mainstream or complementary therapy you feel may help. There is a guide to finding a nutritionally orientated doctor at the end of this book. Use it.

The same applies in the case of seeking a medical specialist. Be aware, however, that changing specialist is much more difficult, and often far less appropriate. In such an instance, it may again be sensible to use a nutritionally orientated doctor as a 'go-between' if your specialist does not see eye to eye with you on the issue of naturopathy, homeopathy or other approaches.

While non-medical health professionals may be the best people for certain aspects of your treatment, there is a need to keep all involved fully informed of your total medical condition if it is at all complicated. You may encounter bias, but since medical specialists are the most likely professionals to be overseeing treatments with the greatest risk of complications and side effects, then they must be fully informed of other treatments so as to assess risks and act accordingly.

Enough said. Let us turn to investigating simple ways of treating dysfunction and disease that you can implement on your own, or at least use as a reference if seeking help from an appropriate health professional, particularly if you fall into the listed categories of concern.

DYSFUNCTION	DISEASE EXAMPLES
Gastrointestinal Dysfunction	Inflammatory Bowel Disease (Crohn's, Ulcerative Colitis), Irritable Bowel Syndrome, Coeliac Disease, Peptic Ulcers, Obesity Other systems disease secondary to malabsorption
Cardiovascular (and Cerebrovascular) Dysfunction	Angina, Myocardial Infarct, Congestive Heart Disease, High Blood Pressure, Stroke, Peripheral Vascular Disease
Respiratory/Airways Dysfunction	Emphysema, Asthma, Sinusitus, Hay Fever
Insulin Resistance	Diabetes Mellitus Diseases related to Cardiovascular Health, Polycystic Ovarian Syndrome Disease, Depression
Hormone Dysfunction	Endometriosis, Hormone Linked Cancers, Polycystic Ovaries, Breast Cysts, PMT Post Natal Depression
Neurotransmitter Dysfunction	Alzheimer's, Parkinson's, Anxiety, Depression, Autism, ADHD, Other Psychological Disorders
Bones, Joints and Muscles Dysfunction	Osteoporosis, Osteoarthritis, Myofascial Trigger Points, Rheumatoid Arthritis/Ankylosing Spondylitis
Immune System Dysfunction	Autoimmune and Hyperreactive Disorders such as Asthma, Rheumatoid Arthritis, Psoriasis and Eczema
Cellular Dysfunction	Chronic Fatigue Syndrome, Fibromyalgia, and almost all other diseases

2

Can Food Be Thy Medicine?

It is often argued that 'super' foods can act as natural medicines, aiding your return to a state of optimal health. Dairy for osteoporosis, blueberries for the brain, seaweed for thyroid metabolism, for example.

But can specific foods actually be used as medicines to treat specific cellular, organ or system dysfunctions or diseases?

The answer is simple. It depends on the particular dysfunction and/ or disease and the time frame in which you wish to see change.

Let us explain. Firstly, all natural approaches to health involving herbs and nutrients work in a similar manner to how most prescription medicines work. Most prescription medicines do not work through an all pervasive mass action due to the presence of chemicals in the tablet. Instead, drugs are most effective when targeting specific cellular activity, coercing natural processes into working towards a healthier body state. Usually this activity results from the interaction of the active ingredient in the drug with a receptor within the pertinent area in which we want the drug to act.

From this, we can argue one simple fundamental point supporting the use of natural medicines for disease. If a drug can work in such a way, so can natural medicine, be it a nutrient or herb. Perhaps not by stimulating a receptor directly, but through the creation of the body's own natural neuropeptides, neurochemicals or hormones that are intended to do the same job.

There have to be relevant neurochemicals in the body to respond to these receptors, otherwise these receptors would be irrelevant, and they obviously are not. We just need to know how to stimulate their natural creation. The only reasonable exception to this argument is when genetic abnormalities exist such that appropriate neurochemicals or protein strands can not be naturally created. However, this is generally an exception, and far from the rule in most chronic disease states.

In fact, when you are in a state of optimal health this is what is happening 100 per cent of the time. You are supplying your body with a satisfactory level of key nutrients and appropriate stimulation through balanced activity as required for good health. Hopefully you are also building up a reserve of nutrients as an insurance policy against future ill health. For instance, the storage of calcium and magnesium in your bones and amino acids in your muscle bulk in order to prevent osteoporosis. Meanwhile, you are avoiding the accumulation of toxins within your system, ensuring that they do not approach critical levels bordering on dysfunction.

And as long as you are following healthy living principles (and do not have a genetic susceptibility) all this can be provided from your food.

But what if (consciously or unconsciously) your body has lapsed into a state of dysfunction or disease, either through poor lifestyle choices, inadequate nutrient intake or genetic susceptibility?

First of all, Step Number 1, is of course to institute non-specific lifestyle changes as described in the first half of this book. You should be doing this whether or not you choose to use food, supplements or prescription medicine. Not only to treat the dysfunction or disease you know about, but as a preventative health measure, and to treat whatever else you don't know about. Remember, singular dysfunctions can lead to multiple potential disease pathways (now or in the future) so there may be 'something' lurking unseen in your Mindbody. Furthermore, cellular health throughout the body requires fundamentally similar nutrient requirements. If dysfunction arises as a result of nutrient insufficiency, there is every reason to suspect you are at increased risk of dysfunction in another system as well.

But what if general measures aren't enough? Will specific foods help specific problems?

Yes, to a point, but there is a limit to how much they will help based once again on our simple understanding of how medicines work.

Remember, whether food, herb or medicine, it is the active ingredient in a food that matters. What we need from our food is a sum of nutrients that will return natural function to our biochemical pathways. We need enough of whatever we require to support the natural creation of protein chains, neurochemicals and so on required for health. Not just to the area of dysfunction, but the whole body.

It is, in fact, the whole body that is experiencing insufficient nutrition, even if it seems only to be a particularly susceptible system that needs attention. This system is simply our breakdown point, our Achilles heel, perhaps owing to genetics or some other predisposition.

Now let us look at what this means in reality using a practical example. In our practice one of the most common nutritional deficiencies identified is magnesium deficiency. Presentations of this deficiency may include musculoskeletal symptoms such as generalised muscle aches and pains, calf and foot cramps, restless legs, eyelid twitches, heart palpitations and an inability to relax. Now 250 milligrams of elemental magnesium twice daily effectively and quickly resolves these symptoms 90 per cent of the time. Note that this is not a recommended daily intake level for ongoing maintenance, rather this is a short-term treatment dosage administered to overcome insufficiency due either to insufficient intake, malabsorption or increased loss.

What if we were to treat this condition through selectively choosing high magnesium foods? Let's look at getting 500mg of magnesium from a single food source. This would mean eating in a day:

- 200g (6½oz) of curry powder (about 40 teaspoons)
- 750g (1½lb) of figs
- 750g (1½lb) of artichoke
- 750g (1½lb) of chocolate
- 500g (1lb) of spinach
- 500g (1lb) of espresso coffee
- 200g (6½oz) of salted peanuts
- 500g (1lb) of bread
- 1½kg/3lbs of steak
- 1¼kg/2lbs 8oz of egg
- 750g (1½lb) of parmesan cheese

And that is assuming effective digestion.

What about choosing a few foods to get the active dosage needed, spreading the intake? Even then you'll still be eating, for example, 20 grams of curry powder, 3 eggs, 125 grams of figs, 125 grams of artichoke, 100 grams of spinach, a pizza base, ¼ kilogram of beef strips and a 50 gram chocolate bar filled with 25 grams of nuts and 5 cups of coffee. That's one very heavy pizza with dessert. What else are you going to eat today?

So you are highly unlikely to consume this level of magnesium in a single day if only focusing on a single, or small number, of magnesium rich foods.

What is in turn demonstrated by this example is that you are also unlikely to achieve fast results from a single food when supplementing for magnesium. You're simply not going to get the dosage that will generally be effective in overcoming the symptoms listed. Not, at least, in the short term. And what holds true for magnesium holds true for most nutrients.

Yet you may achieve the same result slowly, if you are prepared to wait for a more reasonable time frame for magnesium to re-accumulate in your body from food sources. After all, chances are you have accumulated your nutrient deficit slowly, so this is only natural. Therefore it might take 9 to 12 months or more, but it is possible. So here's the important question.

How long are you willing to wait for the changes you desire?

And ironically, how much money are you willing to spend on magic foods, that may be better spent on a quality, fast acting supplement?

The argument stretches a little further, however. As we shall find in further discussions, nutrients work together. You generally do not only need magnesium, you also need B Group vitamins that work hand in hand with magnesium. So if you want an effective super food to work on biochemical grounds, it is also going to need to contain a relevant sum of B Group vitamins. If you're lucky, this may already be in your magnesium rich super foods. However, for argument's sake, let's say the nutrient required is Vitamin B6. This is available predominantly from animal meats, nuts and seeds. So now you'll need to limit your super food group even further, and get even more specific on your food choices.

One kilogram of animal meats and 200 grams of nuts and seeds. How are your saturated fat levels doing?

It is also important, however, to consider that you need to respect certain proportions between different nutrients in your body. For instance, you should try to keep a two-to-one ratio of calcium to magnesium intake. Now, if you eat a balanced diet you will do this naturally. Yet, if you choose to eat one food at a super dosage, this is unlikely to happen. Unless you yet again become even more specific in your food choices. In the above example, your calcium to magnesium ratio is going to be hard to achieve with a single super food dosage (and if you throw in the need for Vitamin B6, you are going to be living on nuts and seeds alone).

In fact this is what modern dietary recommendations risk doing in over emphasising calcium from dairy products (or imbalanced supplements) for the treatment of osteoporosis. Why? Because the calcium to magnesium ratio of dairy products is usually eight to one or greater, so you need to do a lot of compensating with magnesium rich foods to accommodate for high dairy intake, particularly since magnesium is equally important in the prevention and treatment of this condition.

So where does this leave your search for super foods?

Yet again where we started.

Eat a wide range of natural foods in moderation.

You can choose to eat certain foods in relatively higher quantities. But the key is in the word 'relative'. As long as your choices do not destabilise your otherwise balanced diet. And as long as higher quantities do not have negative effects of their own. For instance, as already mentioned, increasing meat consumption to attain higher levels of Vitamin B6, iron or zinc should not come at the risk of increased saturated fat intake. And the increased consumption of deep sea oily fish should take into account the unfortunate environmental risk of increased intake of dioxins, PCBs and other toxins.

So you can focus on particular food groups for added nutrient effect. But the key is, only if in balance. Remember that the results of using food as medicine will take time. Usually months or years, if the condition you are experiencing is significant enough to be providing you with discomfort. Simply put, you're talking the long-term.

On the other hand, for long-term benefit, food should ultimately become your medicine. Once treatment has stabilised your nutrient levels, and hence function, your Healthy Eating Plan, along with exercise and mental hygiene, should simply be what sustains your health. **This ultimately is the baseline for achieving optimal health. No need for supplements, no need for medicines.**

There may be reasons why you are unable to achieve this, particularly if you have already sustained permanent damage from a disease process (see the next chapter for other reasons), but this should be your long-term aim all the same. To have healthy eating and living take over from any short-term intervention you choose, be it nutritional supplements, medication, or even surgery.

Are there any exceptions to this argument?

Are there foods that can work over the short-term as medicines?

Yes, there are. Where there exists an active ingredient within a food that can effectively cross the gut wall and remain active. If this active ingredient can work within a swift time frame it can be a medicine in its natural organic state. The most prevalent examples are usually fresh herbs such as coriander, garlic or ginger (which are therefore used a lot in Ayurvedic cooking). Unsweetened grapefruit used for particular liver detoxification pathways, and 100 per cent cranberry juice for prevention of urinary tract infections are other examples.

Another area in which foods can work swiftly and independently is through directly affecting the balance and health of the gastrointestinal tract (e.g. unsweetened probiotic containing foods such as kefir, 100 per cent prune juice as a laxative). This is because the gut directly absorbs its own nutrients without the need to disperse them equally about the body. Furthermore, foods containing antifungal, antiviral or antibacterial qualities such as garlic are directly able to attack these micro-organisms in the gut prior to being broken down by digestion.

Enzyme containing foods such as pawpaw also help the body's own enzymes absorb foods, again prior to being deactivated by the digestive process.

Finally, we have also highlighted the opposite effect, that the removal of foods can also have a swift effect on a person's signs and symptoms, if they in fact have an intolerance to that food. This is worth remembering, and is covered elsewhere (see Food Intolerances).

So the answer to the question of whether or not to depend solely on whole foods as your medicine comes back simply to the extent of dysfunction and the time required for healing. Are you willing to wait the likely time frame for the required treatment effects to accumulate when using food as a medicine, as well as accepting the increased likelihood that in this subtle approach, nutrient levels are likely to be imbalanced and therefore contribute to other potential problems?

Remember that the following is generally, although not always, true:

- Prescription drugs, if they work, usually take a few hours to days.
- Supplements, if they work, usually take a few weeks to months.
- Foods, if they work, generally take a few months to years.

On the other hand:

- Side effects are highly unlikely for foods.
- Less likely for supplements used responsibly.
- And more likely for prescription drugs.

So the choice really is yours, all things considered. However, the Healthy Eating Plan we have outlined will take you 90 per cent of the way food is going to get you anyway.

Why?

Because the spread of foods recommended (including fresh herbs) will cover you for the majority of your nutrient needs.

After which a few selectively chosen and well considered foods in moderation may take you the rest of the way. If you want to know which foods and why, there are plenty of opinions in your bookstore, but here is a summary of current views for you to begin with.

FUNCTIONAL FOODS AND WHOLE HERBS

The following foods are considered to have health benefits in addressing particular disease or dysfunctional states. For foods containing high levels of specific nutrients, see Section 3, Chapter 6, 'The Quest for Magical Foods'.

Antioxidant rich foods	See above for Vitamins A, C, E, Selenium, Zinc and Lipoic Acid rich foods
Cellular Detoxification	Garlic, Sulphur foods, Antioxidant rich foods
Foods reputed to be Cancer Protective	Fibre rich foods (see above), Antioxidant rich foods, Green Tea, Turmeric, Broccoli, Cauliflower, Cabbage, Brussels Sprouts, Lettuce (Variety), Leafy Green Vegetables, Mustard Seeds, Eggplants, Beetroot, Apples, Pineapples, Banana, Pawpaw, Cherries, Garlic, Ginger, Onion, Yoghurt, Vegetable Juices
Anti-Nausea	Ginger, Raspberry Leaf Tea
Anti-Microbial	Garlic, Ginger, Oregano, Coriander, Liquorice, Rhubarb, Onion, Rosemary, Turmeric, Horseradish, Honey, Thyme, Cinnamon
Digestion	Unsweetened Yoghurt, Enzyme containing foods, Peppermint, Lemon Juice, Angostura Bitters and Apple Cider Vinegar (HCl secretion), Fibre rich foods, Dandelion Tea (Bile secretion)
Laxative	Liquorice, Liquorice Tea, Fenugreek, Fibre foods, Olive Oil
Diarrhoea	Oats
Diuretic	Celery

Liver Support	Artichoke, Asparagus, Garlic, Sulphur foods, Moderate levels of high quality proteins, Antioxidant rich foods (Turmeric), Grapefruit (if high Phase 1 Detoxification), Organic Fruit and Vegetables in general
Cardiovascular Support	Garlic, Ginger, Omega-3 Fat Foods, Antioxidant rich foods, Lentils and Beans, Apples, Bananas, Grapes, Eggplant, Carrot, Broccoli, Onion, Capsicum, Oats, Lecithin Granules, Alfalfa Sprouts, Magnesium rich foods, Fibre rich foods
Cerebrovascular Support	As for Cardiovascular Support plus Berries (especially blueberries, cherries, blackberries), Coffee
Homocysteine control	B Group, Folate and Magnesium rich foods
Anti-Clotting	Ginger, Garlic, Omega-3 Fat rich foods
Pro-Clotting (Bruising)	Vitamin K rich foods
Blood Pressure	Garlic, Ginger, Onions
Respiratory Health	Antioxidant rich foods, Garlic, Horseradish, Fenugreek Herb Tea
Insulin Sensitivity	Carrots, Oats, Beans and Lentils, Fibre rich foods, Lecithin granules, Omega-3 Fats rich foods, Magnesium, Chromium and Zinc rich foods, Coffee
Sex Hormone Balance	Broccoli, Cauliflower, Cabbage, Beans (Soy Beans), Sage, Fennel, Yam, Oats
Thyroid Support	Iodine, Selenium and Zinc rich foods
Neurotransmitter Health	Quality Essential Amino Acids, Magnesium rich foods
Anti-Stress	Lemon Grass, Sage, Chamomile Tea, High magnesium foods, High Vitamin C foods
Sleep Tonic	Chamomile Tea
Bones	Foods rich in both Calcium and Magnesium, Boron, Manganese and Vitamin K, Beans and Lentils, Nuts and Seeds

Joints	Sulphur rich foods, Omega-3 Fat rich foods, Vitamin C rich foods plus other Antioxidant rich foods, Seafoods including Shellfish
Muscles	Magnesium and B Group rich foods
Pain Relief	Cayenne Pepper, Nuts and Seeds
Anti-Inflammatory	Garlic, Ginger, Turmeric, Onions, Apples, Omega-3 rich foods, Liquorice, Pineapple, Pawpaw
Eyes	Antioxidant, Bioflavonoid and Carotene rich foods
Skin	Antioxidant Vitamin, Biotin, Bioflavonoid, Omega-3 Fats, Carotenoid and Zinc rich foods
Hair	Biotin and Silicon rich foods

3

To Supplement or Not To Supplement?

Here goes the simple argument. All of our vitamins and minerals can be obtained from our foods. It doesn't matter what your circumstances, this is the case. Our foods contain everything as long as we have a balanced diet. Besides, when was the last time you saw anybody with scurvy (Vitamin C deficiency), rickets (Vitamin D deficiency) or beri-beri (Vitamin B1 deficiency)? Our foods are perfect and all is good in the world. In fact, take too much of a vitamin or mineral supplement and the result can be toxic, even fatal. They can even interact with your proper medication so that you get even worse side effects.

Case closed. Don't take vitamins and mineral supplements.

Sorry, the defence wants to speak. First of all, those last two arguments can be simply rebutted. If you don't want to suffer the side effects of excess vitamin and mineral intake, don't take too much (like you wouldn't of any of your medications that also have side effects). And if you don't want your vitamins and mineral supplements to interact with the drugs you are taking, ask your doctor or pharmacist to check the possible interactions and/or consult a drug-nutrient-herb interaction textbook as necessary.

So that's the simple question of safety out of the way.

Now to arguing the case that nutritional supplements have a place in maintaining your health.

Take the 'I see no scurvy' argument. Let's have a quick look at some of what Vitamin C does in your body. It's an antioxidant. It helps red blood cell development. The growth of teeth and bones requires Vitamin C. It builds connective tissue. Detoxifies toxins. Helps excrete heavy metals. Improves iron absorption. Improves immunity. Helps your sperm wiggle. Maintains your cell membranes. Has a role in adrenal and ovarian function. Helps fight cancer and prevent cholesterol from forming atherosclerotic plaque. Aids wound healing. And that's just a few functions of Vitamin C.

Now scurvy is the extreme of Vitamin C deficiency. However, an inadequacy of Vitamin C may lead to many and varied effects prior to causing scurvy. Simply look at the varied functions of Vitamin C as listed above and imagine what would happen if each of these areas experienced an insufficiency.

Here are two examples for you to consider.

What happens to your risk of succumbing to the common cold when you have low Vitamin C levels? It increases. Why? Because Vitamin C supports the immune system. No scurvy, but ill health may still result.

More serious still, what happens to your need for Vitamin C when you have cancer? Vitamin C helps fight tumours, so suddenly it is very helpful to have more than the average daily requirement. After all, you have more cancer cells than the average person! In fact, some nutritional doctors will use large doses of Vitamin C intravenously in such a situation, much larger doses than you can get from your fruit and vegetables or even oral nutritional supplementation. Again, no scurvy, but definitely a need for more Vitamin C.

And what is true of Vitamin C equally applies to the many and varied roles of almost all vitamins and minerals the body requires. Unfortunately, modern medicine often overlooks this fact in its arguments against vitamin supplementation, by being fixated to an extent on the view that disease is a polarity, not a continuum. You either have a disease when you reach a critical point reflecting a definable set of signs and symptoms, or you are well, nothing in between. You either have scurvy, and hence Vitamin C deficiency, or your Vitamin C levels are perfect.

But you know better. There is a continuum from feeling great to feeling good, feeling average to feeling down, feeling fatigued to feeling sick enough to go to the doctor, and only then does the doctor consider whether or not you have a disease. But what do you want to feel?

That's so simple.

Great. Vibrant. Sexy.

What does that mean in terms of health maintenance?

It might be the case that Mr, Mrs or Miss Average who is exercising well (but not too much, as this increases your free radicals and hence need for antioxidants), eating a healthy diet (which may need to be organic), is not stressed (because stress depletes your Vitamin C, B Group vitamins and magnesium), does not have a diagnosable disease (whether known or unknown), doesn't smoke (more free radicals, more antioxidant load) or use medication (including the contraceptive pill), may be getting all they require from their food (assuming, of course, the soil the food was grown in had the minerals in it in the first place, regardless of it being organic) …

But are you Mr, Mrs or Miss Average as described above? Let's consider, for a moment, what might be putting you at risk of specific nutrient deficiency.

- An Unhealthy Eating Pattern (whether or not you know it). Are you getting the spread of foods suggested by the Healthy Eating Plan in this book?
- A Fad Diet being any diet that takes you away from an even spread of foods across all food groups. Remember, you need fat soluble vitamins, so guess what happens to these, for example, on a very low fat diet?
- You have poor digestion caused by such various factors as having food intolerances, enzyme insufficiency or genetic differences that lead to inadequate food absorption.
- You drink more than the recommended level of alcohol. There goes some of your B group vitamins, Vitamins A and C, zinc, magnesium and calcium.
- Do you smoke? This irritates your digestive system and demands a much higher intake of Vitamin C and other antioxidants to accommodate for the toxic burden faced by the lungs, as well as the need to help scavenge mutating cells.
- Do you overcook your food? There goes much of its goodness; B group vitamins, Vitamins C and E. Do you prepare your salads in the morning or eat pre-cut salad bar items? Same effect. Do you eat breads? Baking takes out a whole host of nutrients due to the high temperature required.
- Are you on antibiotics? There go the good bugs as well as the bad. And these good bugs aren't just passengers, they actually help with

absorption of various vitamins and minerals through the stomach and intestine, as well as additional roles in immune system management.

- Taking laxatives? This may take out much of your capacity to absorb the fat soluble vitamins K, E, A and D, as well as minerals such as potassium and magnesium.
- Are you a teenager, a pregnant woman (particularly if on your second or third closely timed pregnancy), elderly, an athlete or heavy labourer? Each of these age groups/lifestyle factors require increased nutrient demands, and if you are unable to accommodate for this, your nutrient levels will decline.
- Are you stressed? It doesn't matter the source, you are in need of increased nutrient support from the B vitamins, magnesium and Vitamin C.
- Do you take the oral contraceptive pill? You're in particular need of Folic Acid, but also a whole host of other nutrients diminished by the pill.
- Do your foods come from an area of intensive farming? Or even an area in which the soils are naturally depleted of certain minerals? (magnesium in the East Coast of Australia, selenium in New Zealand).
- Are you taking any other medications not listed here, and do you know what this is doing to your nutrient balance? For instance, the Statin drug group used to combat the negative effects of cholesterol also reduces Coenzyme Q10, a vital nutrient that naturally protects against all things related to heart disease and energy. Ironic, isn't it? This is not to say, don't take your Statins, but you may need to accommodate by taking Coenzyme Q10. Note that this effect is not an isolated occurrence but relatively common. It certainly pays to know how your medication is affecting your nutrient intake.
- And what are your specific disease requirements? You need to see a nutritional practitioner to establish this for the list of disease to nutrient needs is long and varied. Needless to say, we have already

given the example of Vitamin C and cancer, but the rationale for supplement use is far more complicated than this, so again, see a practitioner for this level of care.

✦ And lastly, how do you simply differ to the next person genetically? Are you as efficient as the next person in digesting nutrients? And what influence does that have on your need for nutrients?

So, what should you supplement?

This is where it gets complicated. Look at all the individual factors we have listed that affect what vitamins and minerals you may or may not need to supplement. It's certainly obvious that you are likely to be different to the next person. This is why trying to argue the case for or against nutritional medicine based upon simply taking a multivitamin is farcical. Multivitamins are useful as a general insurance against nutritional inadequacy, but certainly will not be adequate when it comes to matching your individual requirements, if in any way your particular circumstances vary considerably from the average.

It's like telling a gardener he can only tend your garden with a lawn mower and nothing else, but then asking him to manicure the lawn, edge the pavements, weed the rock wall, prune the trees and fix the broken roof on the pergola!

Another important message is this: vitamins and minerals do not work in isolation. They work in functional groups and within balanced parameters.

Take an antioxidant in isolation. Let us use Vitamin E as an example. At low doses Vitamin E has an anti-oxidant effect (keeping it simple, an antioxidant is a chemical that neutralises the effects of oxygen linked toxins created by normal body processes such as breathing and exercise. Conversely, substances that are increased by toxic states are called free radicals).

The anti-oxidant dosage effect of Vitamin E grows until reaching its most beneficial intake at 400–500 IU. After which, the effects of supplementation reverses, and Vitamin E actually encourages oxidation at levels above 500 IU (becomes pro-oxidant).

Given this knowledge, what should be our response to Vitamin E supplementation? Should we avoid taking Vitamin E because it eventually becomes toxic, as some would suggest? No. You don't stop taking a prescription drug because it eventually becomes toxic, you just follow the guidelines and take the recommended dose. So in regard to our example, if you take Vitamin E supplements, don't take more than 500 IU. This isn't rocket science!

But the interesting question is, why does Vitamin E become toxic? Vitamin E becomes toxic because it works as part of a chain reaction. To make this chain work you need a full complement of nutrients to continue the chain. Otherwise, once Vitamin E has done its work, there is nothing else left to finish the job. And so the process stops halfway, at the point at which Vitamin E has done its job, pooling up the products of its function.

Think of a car factory where the Vitamin E puts the axle on. You can put a lot of axles on cars but if there are not enough people to fit the tyres thereafter, sooner or later the process line is going to back up and break down. Nothing wrong with the Vitamin E, it's doing its job. The problem is that Vitamin E is only one part of the chain.

Simple, isn't it? Except that many professionals studying the effects of vitamin E simply note that Vitamin E eventually gets toxic, and so you shouldn't use it.

Simple solution. When using an anti-oxidant supplement, respect the whole chain. Use as broad a spectrum of anti-oxidants as you can achieve in balanced amounts. Not just Vitamin E, but other anti-oxidants as well, including but not exclusively Vitamin A, betacarotene, Vitamin C, Vitamin E, the amino acid cysteine, Coenzyme Q10, lipoic acid and herbs such as garlic (Allium) and gingko, along with the anti-oxidant supporting minerals, selenium, manganese and zinc.

The same is true of B group vitamins. Most B group vitamins work together in a team. They're not a perfectly happy family, however, even if they work together to make your body one. Like all families, they compete at the table and the higher dosage wins. So individual B group vitamin use can be counterproductive, depleting the B group vitamins you are not supplementing for. Therefore, you need to use a broad spread B group vitamin supplement with magnesium for supplementation to be optimally effective. Again, another reason why simple single nutrient studies are not necessarily smart ones.

What about mineral intake? Here, too, balance is sensible. We need to respect the ratios between the minerals we consume. We need calcium for osteoporosis. So should we megadose on calcium (tablet, dairy)? No. Why? Because in order to build bone we need more than calcium. First and foremost, we need to have at least half as much magnesium as any calcium dosage. You will also need boron, manganese, Vitamin K, zinc, a small dose of copper to keep the ratios right (with zinc), and, of course, Vitamin D. There you have it, a balanced supplement for osteoporosis, rather than a megadose of calcium chalk!

Simple? Not necessarily at this point. But here is where nutriceutical and even pharmaceutical companies are starting to get wise. The days of needing to take ten pills from eight different bottles are numbered. Nutritional supplements are increasingly being tailored to meet the needs of specific groups, and while this is not 100 per cent personalised supplementation, (and this, too, is becoming available) it's certainly better than it used to be.

This is where you will need to look at your lifestyle and health position and make informed choices. The remainder of this book is dedicated to this cause.

Otherwise, you could also seek professional advice from a nutritionally orientated practitioner or doctor. Even if you are healthy but have considered it worthwhile to take supplements (other than a simple multivitamin), it is worthwhile seeing a health practitioner. Why? Think about it. If you are going to be taking supplements for the next few years, how much are you going to spend? Compare this to the cost of one or two visits to a nutritionist, naturopath or nutritional doctor to make sure that what you spend is going to do the right job. Better than spending a lot of money on inappropriate supplements, or worse still, megadoses that are likely to lead to toxicity. Either way, you will need to find a credible practitioner or do lots of reading, especially if you are far from Mr, Mrs or Miss Average.

Irrespective of whether you suffer from dysfunction or disease or whether you're simply optimising your health, here are some general rules for supplement intake:

- Always remember, supplements are not a replacement for a healthy diet. They are to be used in addition to a Healthy Eating Plan, not to substitute it.
- First and foremost, tell your doctor you are taking supplements, even if they don't want to hear. A doctor needs to know what you are taking in case it clashes with the medicine he or she wishes to give you.
- Purchase from a reputable source and company that ensures dosages are balanced and consistent between formulae.
- If you have chosen not to consult a health professional, ask for advice from the salesperson but take into account their own potential biases towards products and health approaches.
- Be wary of single nutrient dosages. Most nutrients need the support of cofactors to be effective. As already noted, balanced relationships exist between the antioxidants, the B group vitamins, calcium to magnesium (2:1 ratio), zinc and copper (10:1 ratio), to name but a few relationships that should be respected.
- Check your food allergies and intolerances. If you have extreme allergies, be aware that many supplements (and some prescription drugs) contain wheat (gluten), dairy (lactose), sugars, soy etc. The health implications of exposure to even small doses of these allergens are extreme, particular if you experience anaphylactic reactions. Commonplace drugs like thyroxine (for hypothyroidism) and the Pill contain lactose. Some highly lactose-sensitive individuals may need to take this into consideration. If you have a volume related intolerance, this will not be as significant.
- Check that any fish oil supplements, particularly Omega-3 sources (such as salmon), are mercury, PCB and toxin screened during production.
- Know how your vitamins should be stored. Light denatures many supplements making them ineffective. Other supplements including many probiotic formulas need to go in the fridge. Supplements also have use by dates, and these need to be respected.
- Consume supplements as recommended. Many supplements are

required to be taken either with a meal or away from a meal, and sometimes separate to other specific supplements that they compete with.

- Seek advice on the best form of any nutrient to take. Nutrients need to be stabilised in a supplement. The additional substance to which a nutrient is bonded will affect how well it is absorbed during digestion, and how effectively it can be used by different parts of the body. For instance, iron, even when consumed from foods, is not effectively absorbed from plant sources due to binding with the phytates found in these sources. Instead, it is more effectively absorbed from animal sources (hence the risk of iron deficiency in vegetarians despite taking plant based supplements). Magnesium can be delivered in several forms (oxide, aspartate, citrate and orotate, for example). However, while each will be absorbed, different formulae are more effective in supporting cellular and mitochondrial function (citrate and orotate predominately). These two examples highlight an important factor with many supplements; how a nutrient is delivered matters just as much as its dosage.

- Unless specified by a practitioner, do not obsessively use too many supplements. Many problems can be solved by simple solutions, not megadoses. The more bottles, the more complications. Again, look for supplement packages, not single shots.

- Beware of what constitutes a toxic level for any supplement. If taking two or more supplements, check that there is not an accumulated dose for any nutrient included in both, increasing your intake above a toxic level.

- Be aware that toxic levels differ for some life circumstances e.g. pregnancy, and account for this when considering dosage.

Finally, the most important message. You're fooling yourself if you are using supplements to substitute for a poor diet. You need to rely on a Healthy Eating Plan first. Supplementation can only cover for the better known vitamin and minerals in your diet. But there is so much else you can get from food including a wealth of phytonutrients from plant based foods. Therefore you can never ignore your diet, whether or not you choose to supplement.

Remember always ...

Eat Right, Exercise, Enjoy Life ... Then Consider Nutritional Supplements!

The following table is an introduction to key vitamins and nutrients required by the body.

Signs of deficiency are provided in order for you to identify any potential nutrient deficiencies you may be experiencing. **We suggest you highlight any sign of deficiency with a fluorescent marker in order to personalise your understanding of nutrient deficiencies.** You may notice that the same symptom may indicate several possible deficiencies. As explained by the text, this is often due to interrelated functions of various vitamins and minerals as identified by the co-nutrients column.

At this point we strongly advise that you do not jump in and try to rectify any potential nutrient deficiencies you identify. Instead, you should keep what you find in the back of your mind as an indication of what to look for during the remainder of the book. For ultimately, when addressing nutrient inadequacies you should first evaluate any deficiency in relation to both its cause and the subsequent dysfunction. You should also choose food groups (see last chapter) or supplements to address the family of nutrients required, rather than an individual nutrient.

*Professional supervision is essential whenever using more than product directions or if you are taking prescription drugs. Levels are for adult use only.

Investigating Individual Vitamins and Minerals

INVESTIGATING INDIVIDUAL VITAMINS AND MINERALS

	Co-nutrients	Organs/Systems Requiring Nutrients	Signs of Deficiency	Deficiency Supplementation* (General advice Only)	Toxicity Risk
EPA/DHA (Fish oils)	Vitamins A, E, B6, Magnesium, Selenium, Zinc	Heart, Immunity, Nerves, Brain function, Blood vessels, Insulin sensitivity, Skin, Joints, Gastro-intestinal tract	Dry flaky skin on back of arms, Goose flesh on arms, Cold hands/feet, Cracked heels, Dandruff, Pale skin patches	2–9g daily	Not generally a risk of toxicity
Vitamin A	Antioxidants C, E, Coenzyme Q10, Lipoic Acid, Selenium, Zinc	Eyes, Antioxidant, Growth, Immunity, Fertility	Dry flaky skin on back of arms, Goose flesh on arms, Premature greying, Acne, Thickened skin patches, Calf tenderness	2500–10,000IU	>5000 IU during pregnancy, Higher doses under medical supervision, Best taken as Betacarotene
Vitamin B1	B Group, Folic Acid Magnesium, Choline	Energy production, Nerves	Calf muscle tenderness, Restless legs	25–100mg/day in divided 50mg doses if towards latter	>1g

	Co-nutrients	Organs/Systems Requiring Nutrients	Signs of Deficiency	Deficiency Supplementation* (General advice only)	Toxicity Risk
Vitamin B2	B Group, Folic Acid, Magnesium, Iron, Copper	Energy production, Nerves, Eyes	Magenta-coloured tongue	25–100mg/day in divided doses of < 50mg (preferred 25mg dose)	Not toxic
Vitamin B3	B Group, Folic Acid Magnesium, Iron, Chromium, Selenium, Copper	Energy production, Nerves, Blood vessels, Pancreas, Joints	Red, raw tongue, Fissures in tongue, Skin tags	25–100mg daily	Higher doses may cause facial flushing which may be reduced with aspirin
Pantothenic Acid (B5)	B Group, Folic Acid, Magnesium, Chromium, Zinc, Copper	Adrenal gland, Joints, Blood vessels	Premature greying, Thickened skin patches	25–100mg	Toxic in very high dosages
Biotin	B Group, Folic Acid Magnesium, Chromium, Manganese	Nails and hair	Premature greying, Thickened skin patches, Brittle nails	1–2mg	Not toxic

Vitamin B6	B Group, Folic Acid, Magnesium, Iron, Chromium, Zinc, Copper	Energy production, Nerves, Heart health, Blood vessels, Bones, Neurotransmitters, Hormone balance, Immunity	Cold hands/feet, Swelling of feet, Dandruff, Thinning hair, Premature greying, Pale eye lids, Thickened skin patches, Anaemia	50–200mg daily	May be toxic if higher doses. If any pins and needles, reduce dose
Vitamin B12	B Group, Folic Acid, Iron, Vitamin C, E, Calcium, Copper	Energy production, Nerves, Fertility, Blood vessels, DNA	Patchy hair loss, Pale eye lids, Anaemia, Small or enlarged tongue	500–1000mg/day	Non toxic
Folic Acid	B Group, Magnesium, Zinc, Iron, Copper	Heart health, Bones, DNA, Neurotransmitters, Hormone balance, Pregnancy, Blood cells	Thinning hair, Premature greying, Pale eye lids	500–1000mg/day	Rarely toxic if combined with Vitamin B12
Vitamin C	Antioxidants A, E, Coenzyme Q10, Lipoic Acid, Selenium, Zinc	Antioxidant, Immunity, Bones, Heart health, Blood vessels Clotting, Eyes, Fertility, Wound healing, Hormone balance, Liver detoxification	Scalloping tongue, Bleeding gums, Mouth ulcers, Dry flaky skin on back of arms, Thinning hair, Premature greying, Skin tags, Red skin spots, Stretch marks, Poor healing	250g to bowel tolerance, which will depend upon how deficient you are	Cease if get diarrhoea, the body's way of telling you to stop

	Co-nutrients	Organs/Systems Requiring Nutrients	Signs of Deficiency	Deficiency Supplementation* (General advice only)	Toxicity Risk
Vitamin D	Vitamin B3, Vitamin K, Boron, Calcium, Magnesium, Manganese	Bones, Teeth	Anterior thigh pain	400–2000 IU/day	>3000 IU over long term therefore limit below this
Vitamin E	Antioxidants A, C Coenzyme Q10, Lipoic Acid, Selenium, Zinc	Immunity, Antioxidant, Heart health, Hormone balance	Dry flaky skin on back of arms, Goose flesh on arms, Stretch marks, Poor healing, Acne scars, Calf tenderness	250–500 IU	May become pro-oxidant at levels >500 IU, particularly if taken in isolation
Vitamin K	Vitamins A, B3, B6, C, E, Coenzyme Q10, Manganese	Clotting Osteoporosis	Bruising, Red eye	200mg/day	No known toxicity
Choline	Vitamin B5, B12, Folic Acid, Inositol	Neurotransmitters, Nerves, Blood vessels, Liver balance	Mouth ulcers	1–10g/day	20g/day leads to fishy smell on breath

Inositol	Vitamin B3, Choline, EPA, Folic Acid	Neurotransmitters, Nerves, Blood vessels, Liver balance	Loss of hair	1–10g/day	Not toxic unless intolerant; may cause gut disturbances
Carotenoids	Antioxidants A, C, E, Coenzyme Q10, Lipoic Acid, Selenium, Zinc	Eyes, Heart Immunity, Antioxidant		20–100mg depending on type	Rarely toxic
Bioflavonoids	Vitamin B6, C, E, Zinc	Antioxidants, Immunity	Bruising, Red eye	Variable depending on type	Rarely toxic
Coenzyme Q10	Lipoic Acid, Vitamin E	Energy production, Heart		100–400mg/day	No known toxicity
Carnitine	Lipoic Acid, Zinc	Energy production, Heart		500–3000mg/day	No known toxicity
Lipoic Acid	Antioxidant Vitamins A, C, E, Coenzyme Q10, Selenium, Zinc	Antioxidant		100–500mg/day	No known toxicity
Calcium	Vitamins A, C, D, K, Magnesium, Boron, Carnotine	Bones, Teeth, Connective tissue, Nerve and muscle, Digestion, Hormones, Neurotransmitters	Cramp, Rib pain (Calcium orotate), Bruising	1000mg/day divided into 3 doses (2:1 ratio to Magnesium)	>3000mg/day

	Co-nutrients	Organs/Systems Requiring Nutrients	Signs of Deficiency	Deficiency Supplementation* (General advice only)	Toxicity Risk
Magnesium	B Group, Vitamin C, D, Boron, Calcium, Potassium	Energy production, Insulin sensitivity, Heart, Muscle relaxation, Hormone control, Bones and teeth, Calcium regulation	Muscle twitches, aches and pains, Cramp, Eye twitches, Heart palpitations, Restless legs, Cold hands/feet	Up to 1000mg/day divided into 3 doses (1:2 ratio with Calcium) (1:1 ratio with Phosphate)	>2g
Zinc	Antioxidants A, C, E, Coenzyme Q10, Lipoic Acid, Selenium	Immunity, Digestion, Fertility, Vision, Brain function, Bones, Growth, Insulin sensitivity	White marks on fingernails, Painful tongue, Mouth ulcers, Cold sores, Skin tags, Dandruff, Poor growth, Premature greying, Stretch marks, Poor Healing, Acne, Cracked ear corners	35-50mg/day (10:1 ratio with Copper)	>150mg decreases immunity 1000mg acute toxicity risk May be toxic over longterm if taken unnecessarily
Chromium	B Group Vitamins, Magnesium, Zinc	Insulin sensitivity, Arteries	Skin tags, Cloudy lenses, Dandruff	100-200mg/day	Higher doses only under supervision
Selenium	Antioxidants A, C, E, Coenzyme Q10, Lipoic Acid, Zinc	Antioxidant, Heart, Immunity, Liver detoxification	Dandruff	100-200mg/day at bedtime	>2mg

Iron	Vitamin B2, B12, C, Copper, Folic Acid, Selenium	Haemoglobin, Heart, Muscle coordination, Energy production	Pale eyelids, Bluish eyes, Flat painful tongue, Horizontal nail lines, Spooned nails, No redness to palm creases when stretched, Brittle hair, Anaemia *Brown hue, loss of body hair may indicate excess e.g. Haemochromatosis (check with doctor)	35mg (elemental), 3 times daily	>100mg/day
Manganese	Vitamin B1, C, K Biotin, Choline, Iron, Zinc	Energy production, Insulin sensitivity, Absorption Vitamins, Blood clotting, Ear function, Thyroid hormone, Bones and joints	Thickened skin patches	15–30mg/day	Rarely toxic unless environmentally induced (mining)
Boron	Vitamin B2, D, Magnesium	Bones		5mg/day	>100mg/day
Iodine	B Group, Vitamin C, Copper, Magnesium, Zinc	Thyroid hormone	Goitre, Thinning eyebrows	250–500mg/day	>2000mg/day

	Co-nutrients	Organs/Systems Requiring Nutrients	Signs of Deficiency	Deficiency Supplementation* (General advice Only)	Toxicity Risk
Silicon		Nails and skin	Brittle skin and nails	20–50mg/day	Unknown Restrict to 50mg
Sulphur		Antioxidant, Liver detoxification, Joints		Not usually supplemented for. Use foods	
Potassium	Vitamin B6, Calcium, Magnesium	Energy production, Heart, Muscle coordination, Growth	Muscle cramps	Preferably not individually supplemented for. Balance with Magnesium and Calcium when supplemented. Use Potassium rich foods instead such as Potassium rich salts.	Too much potassium in supplement form may seriously affect your heart. Check blood levels before supplemental use
Copper	B Group, Iron, Magnesium, Zinc	Bone, Heart	Varicose veins, Premature greying	5mg (1:10 Copper:Zinc ratio)	>250mg Acute. 40mg accumulates copper in the system. Copper is a common environmental excess therefore care should be taken

A general multivitamin and mineral should include

Vitamin A 2500 IU and/or Betacarotene 3–5mg
Vitamin B1 25–50mg
Vitamin B2 25–50mg
Vitamin B3 50mg
Vitamin B5 (Pantothenic Acid) 25–50mg
Vitamin B6 25–50mg
Vitamin B12 20–50ug
Folic Acid 200–400ug
Biotin 50–100ug
Vitamin C 100–200mg
Vitamin D 200–300 IU
Vitamin E 25–50 IU
Vitamin K 50ug (particularly for women)
Calcium (elemental) 50–100mg
Magnesium (elemental) 50–100mg
Zinc 5–10mg
Iron 5mg
Chromium 25–50ug
Selenium 25–50ug
Manganese 1–2.5mg

With additional trace minerals (Copper, Boron, Potassium, etc), Bioflavanoids, Choline and possibly Inositol, plus herbal constituents (usually varies depending upon sex and age bracket).

4

The Place of Medicine

We have already examined health as a continuum, from health to dysfunction and from dysfunction through to disease. Understanding health and illness in this context also places us in a good position to evaluate the treatment continuum.

Contrary to the often antagonistic viewpoints of both conventional medicine and what has long been termed alternative medicine (although 'complementary' medicine is definitely preferred), treatments ranging from food and supplements to surgery, radiotherapy and chemotherapy, exist within a continuum of potentially appropriate interventions. It is important to note this continuum does not exclude physical, psychotherapeutic and even spiritual interventions where appropriate.

All therapies exist with the promise to complement each other, if we choose to widen our perspective regarding medicine to incorporate an integrative viewpoint.

Optimal health comes from combining the best elements of all available therapies. Starting with lifestyle modifications—the fundamental baseline for good health—we should not ignore the potential for supplements to aid our cause, nor should we turn our back on medication when it is needed. Among the fields of mental health, you might need a combination of self initiated emotional investigation, counselling, psychotherapy, psychology or psychiatric medication. Whatever is necessary. The same applies to the physical therapies, be they massage, exercise therapy, physiotherapy, chiropractic, osteopathic or otherwise.

So if you are willing to accept the integration of all potential therapies in order to maximise your care, how do you decide which approach to your personal care is most appropriate?

It is obvious that whatever treatment you choose should work. But this is not, in fact, the first rule of medicine. The first rule is:

First Do No Harm!

When we consider Integrative Medicine from this perspective we can develop clear guidelines for choosing how best to combine therapies. And the simple guidelines can be as easily defined as this:

Minimal Intervention, Maximal Gain, Minimum Side Effects

Ultimately, it will depend upon your state of health as to how you apply these guidelines.

For instance, if I am healthy and experience diarrhoea I might simply choose to do nothing. Perhaps I just ate something bad, and my good health will deal with the circumstances soon enough. If I was a little more proactive, I might consider a combination of consuming oats (soluble fibre) and increasing my fluid intake. If this did not work, I may turn to probiotics, and consider further supplementation depending upon the associated symptoms.

If the condition persisted I might then have a stool culture performed, and depending upon the results, use anti-microbial herbs or an antibiotic, followed up with probiotic rehabilitation. Note that I am now using a specific treatment with side effects (antibiotics) and that I am now minimising these side effects with subsequent therapies (probiotics).

But ultimately, if I discovered I had cancer of the bowel, suddenly I might be willing to consider chemotherapy, radiotherapy and surgery, to save my life. These treatments may be augmented by the use of antioxidant supplements. For example, being aware of serious side effects I might also integrate my care with the use of probiotics, glutamine, ginger, garlic and Vitamin E in an attempt to avoid mouth sores and nausea. I might also change my diet and take a multivitamin or multiple higher dose supplements to overcome some of the nutrient depletions that may arise as a consequence. All of this, of course, in consultation with and between my naturopath and medical doctor and specialist.

What is being highlighted by this example is the continuum of interventions available. Where health is optimal, little needs to be done to finetune it, and so, in turn, little is risked. Yet when health is at risk, our interventions may need to be stronger. It is usually the case that this places us at risk of increasingly likely and serious side effects that should be accounted for and accommodated where possible.

We highlight the necessity here of collusion with a doctor (both general practitioner and consultant specialist) when considering any intervention involving complex prescription medication, chemotherapy, radiotherapy, surgery or other serious intervention.

Why? Because these interventions must be overseen by a doctor in order to ensure serious side effects of treatment are being accounted for and protected against including interactions with other forms of medicine such as nutritional supplementation. **No-one else is licensed to undertake such a role.**

This in turn implies responsibility from your doctor for being aware of the available options for minimising the side effects of any treatment, both within his or her field of expertise (prescription medication) as well as the options available from fellow practitioners, whether in mainstream or complementary fields. At the very least your doctor should know when a complementary treatment may cause risk (through interacting with prescribed medication), while also respecting another practitioner's advice regarding interventions that may contribute to all-round care.

The use of lifestyle modifications, food as medicine, supplementation or any other treatment should therefore not be seen as conflicting with prescribed medication unless proof of adverse or side effects can be established. Furthermore, since such treatment approaches often incur far fewer side effects than most medicines, they should be considered first in the continuum of care, wherever effectiveness has been shown, prior to resorting to stronger medications.

On the other hand, where dysfunction or disease has progressed beyond the capacity for nutritional medicine or any other conventional therapy to provide optimal care, prescription medicine, chemotherapy, radiotherapy or surgery should equally be respected and used until less invasive therapies can once again replace them if possible. This, in turn, implies the need for complementary practitioners to show equal respect to conventional medical practitioners, understanding the place and use of prescription medication.

When prescription medications risk depleting vital and key nutrients, every effort should be made to account for this by supplementation in order to restore the nutrients depleted. When a nutrient can be used to either augment the use of a prescription drug, making that drug more effective (meaning less needs to be used) or can be used to eliminate a side effect of a medication, such use should also be considered.

The table at the end of this chapter indicates how some of the most commonly used drugs interact with the nutritional status of your body. It is meant to highlight the various effects that may occur when drugs and foods, nutrients or herbs are combined. It may come as a surprise to many (particularly those on either side of the conventional versus alternative medicine antagonism) that nutrients and drugs can often be used to complement each other. Whenever possible this should be worked to effect the most beneficial care while respecting the tenet, 'Minimal Intervention, Maximum Gain, Minimal Side Effects'. In summary, the relationship between a drug and food, nutrient or herb may be such that:

- A drug may adversely affect the nutrient status of your body, in which case supplemental nutrients may be required to prevent deficiency.
- A drug may interact with a food, nutrient or herb such that the combination may cause serious side effects. In which case, where the drug is essential to care, the food, nutrient or herb should be withdrawn.
- A nutrient or herb may alternatively be used to diminish the side effects of a drug.
- A nutrient or herb may actually make a drug more effective. This leads to the possibility of the nutrient or herb being used to diminish the required dosage of the drug. However, if this is uncompensated for, the nutrient or herb may instead cause a build up of a medication in the body, leading to toxic levels or side effects.

* A nutrient or herb might also decrease the effectiveness of a drug.

Where prescription drugs are involved you will be under the care of a medical doctor. But it is vital your doctor is aware of how best to negotiate all the above issues, and is interested in understanding the integration of prescription medication with foods, nutrients or herbs, if you are to maximise your health.

Therefore, if you are interested in the minimalist approach to effective medical care recommended in this book, you may need to establish your own 'team' of open-minded and proactive medical practitioners (starting with a doctor and naturopath, herbalist or nutritionist) willing to cooperate in integrating your medical care. Unless, of course, you are attending a nutritionally orientated medical doctor with broad expertise and the time required to thoroughly balance your needs.

Such a team must respect one another and their respective fields of expertise.

Your doctor must be informed regarding all you are doing, but in turn should also be aware or willing to investigate other options you may choose, and how it impacts on the prescription drugs you are taking. On the other hand, complementary medical practitioners must also respect when a person reaches a stage on the health continuum where prescription medications (however serious their side effects) are a necessity, and be willing to work within the parameters that such drugs create.

When you are on prescription medication a need arises to establish a baseline of understanding between yourself, an open-minded doctor, and complementary medical professionals. You should never take matters into your own hands when it comes to adjusting your prescription medication. This is your doctor's role.

Even if your doctor is unwilling to listen to your requests, do not stop taking prescribed medication or, on the other hand, prescribe your own intensive supplement program without consultation.

Instead, consider seeking a nutritionally orientated doctor, or at least a more open-minded conventional doctor willing to expand their knowledge and work with others, and allow this new member of your health team to adjust your care appropriately.

EXAMPLES OF DRUG NUTRIENT INTERACTIONS

The following table is used for example purposes only. No action should be taken in relation to this table unless indicated by a medical doctor. The list is far from complete. A comprehensive review of this subject can be found in: *A–Z guide to Drug–Herb–Nutrient Interaction,* Lininger et al, 1999)

ACE Inhibitors (Treatment for High BP)	Chronic use increases loss of zinc, with related risks to copper due to need for healthy zinc-copper ratio May increase blood potassium levels. Should not use a potassium supplement or salt with ACE inhibitor. Care needs to be taken not to over consume high potassium foods (e.g. bananas, potatoes, avocado)
Salbutamol [Ventolin] (Treatment for Asthma)	Known to reduce plasma levels of Calcium, Magnesium, Potassium and Phosphate. Magnesium is important for smooth muscle relaxation, for which Salbutamol is also taken, thus suggesting a conflicting effect that may need to be supplemented for
Antacids (Aluminium based)	Aluminium based antacids increase the loss of calcium and phosphorous from the body, a long-term risk being osteoporosis
Antibiotics	Depletion of Lactobacillus Acidophilus leading to destabilisation of stomach flora. Need to re-establish probiotics after course of antibiotics Depletion of Vitamin K by destroying friendly micro-organisms that synthesise it Vitamin C may improve the effectiveness of antibiotics Saccharomyces boulardi, a supplemental yeast, may prevent diarrhoea associated with antibiotic use

Chemotherapy Drugs	A wide range of nutrients are at risk of decline during chemotherapy as a result of malabsorption or depletion. Folic acid decreases the effectiveness of Methotrexate (but not other chemotherapy drugs), and in turn is diminished by the use of Methotrexate While controversial, antioxidants are believed to support the use of many chemotherapy drugs Side effects of chemotherapy such as mouth sores (aided by Topical Vitamin E, Betacarotene, Ginger and Glutamine), Diarrhoea (Glutamine) can be aided by nutritional supplementation. Ginger may assist with nausea
Contraceptive Pill	Understood to deplete Vitamins B1, B2, B3, B6, B12, C, Folic Acid, Zinc, Manganese and Magnesium. The associated B6 deficiency has been linked to depression Increases absorption of Calcium, Copper and Vitamin A
Corticosteroids	Known to deplete DHEA and Melatonin, Vitamin A, B6, D and K, Magnesium, Zinc, consequences of which include risk of Osteoporosis Can cause muscle wasting therefore increased protein intake may be recommended Some users need to restrict salt (NaCl) as sodium retention may occur Aloe vera may improve the effects of topical application of Corticosteroids.

Non-Steroidal Anti-Inflammatory Drugs	Some NSAIDS (Ibuprofen, Indomethacin, Naproxin) may cause iron loss and GI bleeding. Therefore iron supplementation may be indicated, but care is needed that an iron supplement does not in turn cause GI upset

Some NSAIDS may cause sodium and fluid retention, therefore salt (sodium based) and salty foods may need to be limited

Copper may make some NSAIDS more effective thus lowering the dosage required

Liquorice extract may decrease the irritation to the stomach caused by NSAIDS |
| Metformin (Diabetes Medication) | May reduce Vitamin B12, Folate and Magnesium (although needs to be confirmed) levels, nutrients important for the Diabetes patient |
| Statin Family (Anti-Cholesterol Drugs) | Statin drugs reduce the levels of Coenzyme Q10 in the body (a nutrient in itself important for heart health). May also deplete Zinc and Vitamin E.

Soluble fibre (e.g. pectin, oat bran) may reduce the absorption of statins |
| Tricyclic Anti-Depressants | Should not be used with St John's Wort

May deplete Coenzyme Q10

Use may be supported by use of most B Group Vitamins |
| Warfarin (Anti-Clotting) | Known to have adverse interactions with a wide variety of vitamins, herbs and even foods high in the associated vitamins including but not restricted to Vitamin C, Vitamin K (for which dietary control of food sources is essential while on this drug), Garlic, Ginger, Pawpaw, Fenugreek, Gingko, Ginseng, Devil's claw, Dong Quai, Red Clover, Sweet Woodruff |

SECTION 5

Investigating Your Personal Supplement Needs

Effective nutritional supplementation simply cannot be applied in a 'one size fits all' fashion. If approached in this way, it is just as likely to succeed as prescribing every patient with heart disease or diabetes a single specific drug and specific dosage only, regardless of age, sex, state of disease or otherwise. No doctor would accept this approach as valid, and nutritional practitioners are no different, even if many of the studies used to argue against the field ignore this.

The following section sets out to highlight the justification for individualised nutritional interventions designed to optimise your health. You can choose to read through each chapter, or identify which chapters are pertinent to you via the questions at the beginning. Also note if you have diseases associated with the particular health system discussed. But do not rush head-first into a supplement regime without first reading through the last section in this book.

We ask you to consult a natural health practitioner or doctor if you have a complex set of health needs. This will be value for money if you are considering a therapeutic trial of supplements, because a few months on the wrong supplements will both waste your time AND cost you the price of a health consultation.

All supplement recommendations in this section are daily dosage recommendations that should be reviewed by a health practitioner.

Where possible, divide dosages across three or more consumption periods (e.g. If taking 3 grams of Omega-3 fish oils take 1 gram morning, lunch and evening)

The information should not, under any circumstance, be used to replace a health professional consultation.

If on prescription medication, you must review any supplement program with your doctor to assess if any contraindications exist between treatments.

This being said, enjoy the journey!!

1

Cellular Health

Cellular health underlies every system in our body. Where widespread symptoms exist without a definitive specific diagnosis, widespread cellular health problems may be suspected. In particular the following questions as related to mitochondrial dysfunction may be pertinent:

1. Do you experience regular episodes of fatigue even after rest? **Yes / No**
2. Do you live with non-specific widespread aches and pains? **Yes / No**
3. Are your muscles generally stiff throughout your body? **Yes / No**
4. Do you experience lethargy, even when motivated towards a personal goal? **Yes / No**
5. Do you find it difficult to focus and feel generally heavy of mind? **Yes / No**

All diagnosable diseases require cellular health support, but specific diseases that are particularly pertinent include:

- ✦ All cancers
- ✦ Functional disorders such as Chronic Fatigue Syndrome, Fibromyalgia, and Myofascial Pain Syndromes
- ✦ Complex disorders such as Alzheimer's Disease, Autism and Attention Deficit Hyperactive Disorder

Please note that this chapter is unavoidably complex as Cellular Health underpins every possible disease process that may occur within our bodies. We shall return to the Simple shortly!

Heart, lungs, kidneys, skin, eyes and testicles. There is one single thing they all have in common: they are made up of cells. And while the primary function of each cell will be ultimately determined by the organ to which it belongs, in the main all cells function in the same way. This means in turn that all cells throughout your body have the same fundamental requirements for healthy survival.

Understanding what these requirements are and why they are important provides a simple lesson as to why adequate nutrition itself is so significant. What we are talking about is simple biochemistry, yet at the same time this is a topic all too frequently overlooked, frowned upon as unimportant or simply taken for granted. It is so often the case that doctors and health practitioners look for some complex cause of disease, or an unchangeable genetic factor, when instead they should first consider the health of the all pervasive and fundamental system of life within our body: the cell.

So what simple functions do all cells have in common?
To name a few:

1. To provide a partially permeable environment that allows the cell to individually survive as an entity. This is the role of the cell membrane, which acts to keep out all but that which is individually required by the cell, whilst still allowing the entry of glucose, amino acids and other nutrients necessary for cellular function.
2. To communicate with the outside world by receiving and releasing signalling chemicals.
3. To understand and respond to the body's messages by in turn building protein chains that correspond to the body's current needs. These protein chains in turn form either further messages (in the form of neuropeptides, hormones etc), building blocks for cellular processes or cell constituents allowing for the multiplication of cells in the body. The body's coding system, DNA, is designed specifically for this process.

4. To provide energy for the above function through the microscopic powerhouses of the human body, the mitochondria.
5. To survive the whole process by detoxifying the side effects of each of the above processes.

Thus each cell in itself can be seen as a living entity not unlike its 'owner', with a brain (DNA), a skin (cell membrane), eyes and ears (receptors on the outside of the cell), a mouth and gut (active and passive transport systems), lungs and heart (mitochondria), a skeletal system (microtubule matrix) and liver (detoxification systems). And each of these 'organ systems' require vital nutrients to work effectively.

How so?

Let's begin with the cell membrane. The cell membrane is a semi-permeable wall meant to only allow selective needs of the cell to penetrate. Within it are contained transport systems that allow this to happen. While some particles naturally penetrate the cell membrane (passive transport),other particles need to be let through by the opening of specific channels (active transport), similar to the way you let yourself into your house with a lock and key. However, in the case of your cell membrane, the lock is a receptor within the membrane that quickly vibrates back and forth in search of specific messenger chemicals, which act as keys.

Therefore, a cell membrane is healthiest when viscous and elastic, allowing this sweeping movement of the receptors.

What is a cell membrane made up of? Largely from fats. And what makes the best cell membranes? Omega-3 essential fatty acids.

You can use other fats but they make for far more rigid cell membranes, affecting all of the functions of the cell wall.

The costs of not having a nice Omega-3 filled cell membrane? That's simple. Impaired receptor function leading to less effective communication between cells. Problems with the transport of essential nutrients across the cell wall. A cell wall that is at greater risk of being infiltrated with athero-sclerosis. And when the cell wall is ruptured, the activation of an excessive inflammatory response during the healing process. This then subsequently causes multiple problems of its own.

Now consider how many disorders/diseases are affected simply by limiting cellular membrane function through an inadequate intake of essential fatty acids. A decrease in intercellular communication (hormones, neurotransmitters), the supply of vital nutrients to cells (sugars and proteins), and a pro-inflammatory environment. Which diseases and dysfunctions might this include?

In fact, you might as well ask which diseases it wouldn't include, whether of genetic origin or not! There simply would be very few diseases not worsened by a poorly functioning cell membrane, from gut to brain and back again.

Why?

Because every cell is affected as every cell has a cell membrane. That's the reality of the importance of Omega-3 Fatty Acids. Eat fatty fish or another dietary source in suitable quantities or use a supplement. It's as simple as that. Omega-6 Fatty acids are also important, but as it is likely you are getting these from your modern-day diet, which in most cases is Omega-6 dominant, we will not argue as strongly for their case. If you do have doubts about your intake, however, you may consider an Evening Primrose Oil supplement if indicated by a practitioner.

CELL MEMBRANE HEALTH

Omega-3 Oils	(EPA/DHA)	2 to 4 grams daily (Maintenance dose)
		4 to 9 grams daily (Treatment dose)

What about the cellular transport systems of our cell wall? Are they affected by nutrient intake, and if so, what are the consequences?

Let's use the example of the transport of glucose into cells. This is discussed in detail in relation to Insulin Resistance in a later chapter, but here is a brief overview. The key that allows sugar into your system is insulin. The lock is greased by chromium picolinate, magnesium and zinc, among other nutrients. And what happens when the key is not greased effectively?

Insulin Resistance, with its impact on almost every cell of the body. Sugar unable to get into the cell means the outside world bathes in sugar, while insufficient sugars on the inside means cellular fatigue. Again, while different cells are affected in different ways due to their particular transport mechanisms, all are universally affected. Why? Because we are affecting the fundamentals of cellular health through influencing the primary fuels feeding their energy systems, and that means each and every cell in the body.

Furthermore, what of the process of protein transcription and the building of protein chains as takes place in the DNA and beyond? First of all, we need to gather all the building blocks to any given task we give the cell. No different than the local car factory. Don't supply an axle and you won't get a completed car. Don't supply the fundamental building blocks of protein chains (the essential amino acids) and you won't get the final product the cell is meant to build for the body.

Are you getting enough building blocks for your car? Or are you short-changing your DNA by not providing the parts? Your body needs a full complement of amino acids from quality protein sources. This means you must either eat an animal source of protein (meat, fish, eggs, dairy), substitute with a reasonable quantity from the nut and legume/ pulse (bean) group or consume a wide variety of cereal/ grains and vegetables to compensate (far less preferable).

You can consume a quality protein supplement powder if you have increased protein needs (athletes, bodybuilders, those afflicted with long-term diseases that cause malnutrition), or for some reason suspect inadequate quality protein in your diet. This is an insurance policy, and will depend on the quality of the powder that you choose. Where consuming a protein powder you should consider:

- ✦ That all essential amino acids are present and in appropriate amounts.
- ✦ How many carbohydrates are in the supplement. Your needs will vary regarding this. If you are replacing a meal, you may wish for added carbohydrate, with the exception being if you are trying to lose weight. If you are not replacing a meal, but simply choosing to

add quality protein to your diet, choose a protein powder with minimal additional carbohydrates.

- The additional micronutrients added, particularly if used as a complete meal replacement. Many supplements have a full range of multivitamin and minerals included, others may not.
- The source. Ensure it is not derived from or contains food groups to which you are intolerant or allergic.

Protein powders are not essential to good health for most, but they do provide an easy way to gain quality proteins if you miss meals, particularly in the form of quickly made breakfast smoothies.

A PROTEIN POWDER WITH A FULL COMPLEMENT OF AMINO ACIDS SHOULD INCLUDE

Alanine, Arginine, Aspartic Acid, Carnitine, Cysteine, Glutamine, Glutamic Acid, Glutathione, Glycine, Histidine, Isoleucine, Leucine, Lysine, Methionine, Phenylalanine, Proline, Serine, Taurine, Threonine, Tryptophan, Tyrosine, Valine

There is another factor regarding the production of proteins that needs to be taken into account. The creation of proteins in every cell requires the addition and removal of certain chemical groups from a protein chain. Just think of adding and removing links that represent the specific essential amino acids required; it need be no more complicated than this. Unfortunately, this does not always happen effectively and this can result in widespread problems.

Take, for example, the elevation in homocysteine that occurs when a particular biochemical pathway called methylation does not work effectively.

What are the consequences of high levels of homocysteine?

Here's a list for you. Alzheimer's. Heart disease including heart attack. Stroke. Almost all cancers. Diabetes. Rheumatoid arthritis. Osteoporosis. Problems with pregnancy. Hypertension. And this is an abbreviated list. What organs are already included? Brain. Heart. Blood vessels. Digestive tract. Reproductive organs. Joints. Bones. Not much left out, is there, even from our abbreviated list?

Why? Because we are talking about a basic cellular mechanism that is going wrong. And so when cellular health fails, the risk incurred is to almost every system in the body. The outcomes may appear to be in only one system, but that is simply because this is the system in which your body first begins to break down. In simple terms, this is your weak link, your Achilles Heel. Unless you do something about the dysfunction it can result in the accumulation of multiple chronic dysfunctions or disease states instead.

So, how do you avoid excess homocysteine from affecting your body? Provide it with nutrients that will work upon every cell to bring down homocysteine levels. What are they? Vitamin B6. B12. Folate. Supported by Coenzyme Q10 and Fish Oils (see Cardiovascular Health for more information).

So you get the factory in order. No breakdowns and the machines well oiled. But what about the power station down the road? Is it working?

Well, it will come as no surprise that every cell uses the same power organ known as the mitochondria. The mitochondria work by using two key ingredients; energy in the form of carbohydrates (most preferable) and fats (stored energy). If desperate, they will also utilise protein. The most important concept to understand, however, is nothing actually happens to the energy source until it gets to the cell, and predominantly, the mitochondria. The lungs, the heart, the digestive tract, the blood vessels, red blood cells and even the cell membrane are simply transport mechanisms.

The real work takes place in the mitochondria of every cell. Again, the process does not differ whether the cell is in the heart, the kidneys, your big toe or your brain. And if all is going right in the world with mitochondrial function, life's a buzz of energy. However, if there is a nutritional inadequacy that affects one cell, it most certainly has the potential to affect every cell in the body.

So, what key nutrients are required for mitochondrial function?

The nutrients required are those cofactors needed in the mitochondrial energy chain (commonly called the Krebs, TCA or Citric Acid cycle). If these vital nutrients are present, the Krebs cycle produces sufficient energy from the fuels presented. If not, the mitochondria malfunctions whether or not there is sufficient fuel made available to it. And what are these key nutrients? Vitamins B1, B2, B3, B6 and magnesium (in aspartate, citrate or orotate forms).

So if these nutrients are deficient, there is the risk of mitochondrial dysfunction leading to energy crisis. Outcome? Widespread fatigue and a loss of function of most body organs.

So when do we need an increased intake of these nutrients? When we need more energy from our mitochondria. When is this the case? During periods in which the body is put under stress, be the latter of physical, emotional or mental origin, including infectious invasion and traumatic insult. This is further made relevant by the fact that these nutrients are also required for the functioning of our brain's communication signals (see Chapter 8 of this section, 'Neurotransmitter Health'), a system also under strain during periods of stress.

ENERGY AND STRESS NUTRIENTS (TREATMENT DOSAGES)

B Complex consisting of
Vitamin B1	(50mg)
Vitamin B2	(50mg)
Vitamin B3	(50mg)
Vitamin B6	(100mg)
Vitamin B12	(500ug)
Folic Acid	(400ug)
Magnesium	(elemental) 500mg

Supported additionally by
Co-Enzyme Q10 (100-150mg),
Taurine (1g)

Dosages are intended for treatment use (when deficiencies are present) or during stressful periods rather than simple maintenance.

The last universal function of each cell is the need to detoxify its own environment. After all, although detoxification takes place to a large extent in the gastrointestinal tract (preventing external toxins from entering into the system in the first place) and liver (filtering extracellular fluids), each cell is still required to clean up much of its own intracellular environment.

And while it would be fair to blame much of the toxic build-up in our body on the infiltration of toxins from the external world (chemicals, food additives, smoking), even in the perfect environment our body is still required to clean up after itself. Why? Because the natural processes required to exercise, fight stress, cope with excessive exposure to light, the simple act of breathing and burning up sugar, to name just a few natural functions, all lead to the release of what are known as free radicals.

Our energy systems are more like nuclear reactors than solar panels in that they release unstable and reactive particles with the potential to create nasty by-products along with the energy they create. In simple terms, these particles lead to the oxidation of our body. Put another way, our tissues are at risk of rusting away when exposed to these particles, no different to iron when exposed to water. In the body, the pro-oxidant particles or free radicals accumulate through the act of cellular respiration as well as toxic accumulation and, if left unchecked, react upon cellular tissues leading ultimately to tissue degradation and dysfunction.

What diseases are progressed (although not necessarily caused) by free radical damage?

Let's start with atherosclerosis, through the degradation and implantation of oxidised cholesterol in the cell membranes of blood vessels. This condition is further complicated by the resulting inflammatory responses subsequently initiated by the body. As a consequence, there are potential influences on heart disease, hypertension (through the effects of atherosclerosis on our kidney vessels), stroke and peripheral vascular diseases.

All forms of cancer, including skin cancer (as a result of oxidant damage caused by light exposure) and lung cancer (oxidant damage as a result of smoking), are made more likely by poor oxidant protection. Emphysema also, as a result of the free radicals caused by smoking. Macular degeneration. Neurodegenerative conditions such as Parkinson's and Alzheimer's Disease. Most skin disorders.

Yet again, since each and every cell needs to be effective in cleaning up its own toxic environment, an inadequacy in the nutrients required for antioxidant activity can lead to any number and combination of issues depending upon an individual's particular susceptibility and personal choice of poison. For instance, smokers risk placing their lungs at greatest risk, sunbathers their skin, and those with poor dietary and exercise commitments, their blood vessels, with a flow-on effect to heart, brain and so forth. By no means, however, are the risks mutually exclusive; rather they are cumulative. As the antioxidant demand of the body in general grows, so the likelihood of nutritional inadequacy and hence systemic free radical damage. **So how do we support cellular detoxification?**

There are two mechanisms to consider. The neutralisation of free radicals via the antioxidant cascade as typified by protective nutrients such as Vitamins A, C and E (the tocopherols and tocotrienols) and Betacarotene, supported by Lipoic Acid, CoEnzyme Q10, Bioflavonoids (Quercetin, Rutin) and a host of other phytonutrients. Remember what was said in the last chapter; you need a combination of antioxidants rather than single nutrient doses, otherwise the cascade may pool at a toxic point halfway through the process of detoxification.

Most of us also have an enzymatic pathway for detoxification via enzymes with complicated names like superoxide dismutase, glutathione perioxidase, perioxinitrite and metallothionein, which are fed via the amino acids glutamine (or glutathione itself), methionine, cysteine and N-acetyl-cysteine and supported by the minerals magnesium, selenium and zinc (balanced with copper). A little more complicated, but added in order to finish the discussion.

CELLULAR DETOXIFICATION

A broadbased antioxidant supplement (treatment dosages) should include:

Vitamins A (2500 IU), C (1 to 3g), E (250-500 IU), Lipoic Acid (100mg), Betacarotene (30mg), Bioflavonoids (1g) [Quercetin, Rutin], CoEnzyme Q10 (100 -150mg) with the potential for a range of Phytonutrients (e.g Grape Seed, Green Tea etc) and herbs (Garlic, Ginger etc).

Additional support for detoxifying enzymes that may be used under practitioner supervision:

Glutathione (1000mg) OR Cysteine (>200mg), Glycine (>5g) and Glutamine(>500mg)]; Superoxide Dismutase, Methionine (>200mg), N-Acetyl Cysteine (>200mg), Lipoic Acid, 100mg ...supported by Zinc (35-50mg elemental), Selenium (50-150ug elemental) and B Complex plus Magnesium (500mg elemental).

So, where does all this lead? Well, first of all, you already understand why Nutritional Medicine (whether through simple food choices or supplement usage) can be effective in maintaining your health.

When your cell has such broadbased needs as discussed in this chapter, it becomes obvious that you should attempt to consume a wide ranging diet of natural whole foods to supply such needs. This is essential, whether or not you choose to supplement.

Furthermore, if you choose to supplement your diet, it will be better to choose a combination of wide ranging nutrient formulations rather than single nutrient shots. What you choose will depend on what you are willing to spend. The most cost acceptable option is a broad ranging multivitamin. If you are willing to spend more, you might choose a combination of an antioxidant formula, B group with magnesium, Fish Oils (Omega-3) with a probiotic if necessary. Market trends are seeing these formulae combined so that you might be able to get this down to three or even two supplements per day.

Unless ...

You identify patterns of dysfunction from the remaining chapters that indicate a need for specific and personalised supplement approaches. If this is the case, you should consider seeing a nutritionally orientated doctor or other practitioner (naturopath, nutritionist etc) to guide you on your path, particularly if you have reached a state of diagnosable disease, and especially if you are taking prescription medication.

Even if you have no symptoms, it is worth discussing supplements with a practitioner anyway. For to repeat what was said in the previous chapter, if you are going to invest in quality supplements, you might as well pay a little more for effective advice, rather than waste money on the wrong supplements.

2

Gastrointestinal Health

If you regularly experience any of the following, you may have Gastrointestinal Dysfunction (circle as appropriate):

Diarrhoea	Constipation
Abdominal Bloating	Excess Flatulence
Excess Burping	Reflux/Indigestion
Indigestion	Antacids usage
Antibiotic usage	Anti-inflammatory usage
Painful bowels relieved by motions	Specific food irritants
Evacuate faeces >3 times per day	Abdominal Discomfort/Pain
Overly hard or soft stools	Pebble-like stools

Diagnosable diseases specifically involving the gastrointestinal dysfunction include:

- Gastrointestinal Reflux, Peptic Ulcers, Chronic Diarrhoea and Constipation, Inflammatory Bowel Disease, Irritable Bowel Disease, Coeliac Disease
- Many other diseases are exacerbated by Food Intolerances/Leaky Gut e.g. Migraine, Inflammatory Arthritis, Autoimmune Disorders, Asthma/Sinusitis/Hayfever

In addressing gastrointestinal health we are working under an assumption that you have already started to change your dietary habits. In particular, that you have started to undertake a Food Elimination Regime (including an initial trial of probiotics).

Only if you have fulfilled these prior measures and are still having problems with digestion and/or elimination need you consider the following steps.

Let's start with the end, which, when considering the gastrointestinal tract, is often an important place to start. Do you suffer from constipation, diarrhoea or a frequent swing from one to the other? If so, it is important to address this situation first. After all, there is no use cleaning up the system if there is no place for the results to go, that is, if you can't remove the toxins from your body! Or, on the other hand, with diarrhoea, that everything will simply be flushed down the toilet!

Foremost, if your constipation or diarrhoea has been occurring for a long period of time, have you consulted your doctor? Are you certain there is not an underlying medical condition that needs to be resolved? Are there any abnormal changes in your stools that need to be considered? Have you a gastrointestinal bug, and if so, do you need a stool analysis, which might reveal the underlying cause as a parasitical, bacterial or fungal invasion that needs treating, in which case you will need more specific intervention through either medical or herbal medication?

Of even more importance is the presence of blood in your stools. If you detect blood in your stools consult your doctor immediately. This is unchallengeably your first port of call. Do not try and treat this yourself. Often blood is hidden in the stools (occult). A simple stool culture will reveal the presence of any red blood cells besides any evidence of infection.

Otherwise there are a few natural solutions to consider for constipation:

+ Start the day with a glass of warm water with lemon juice. Finish the day with a glass of warm water.
+ Eat natural laxative foods. Figs, prunes (juice), apricots, olive or flaxseed oil and rhubarb.
+ Also eat foods high in fibre; fruits, vegetables, wholegrain breads (if tolerant), raw nuts, seeds and legumes.
+ Keep up the fluids. You definitely need your 8 cups today.
+ Excess coffee often relieves constipation, but can have other side effects, so beware of relying on this.

- Keep walking and exercising.
- Squat to toilet.

Anything happening?

There are a few supplement tricks you can try as well. Most obvious is to use a fibre supplement containing psyllium, guar or similar product, as long as it is an insoluble form of fibre. Aloe vera or slippery elm may also help. Get back on your good quality probiotics. Keep up the fluids. If this doesn't work, try Vitamin C. How much? Fill yourself up to what is called Bowel Tolerance. That is, until you have had so much Vitamin C that your body can no longer absorb any more and you get diarrhoea. In most cases this works. (This is also a good test to show how deficient you may be in Vitamin C. As the deficiency decreases, so will the dose of Vitamin C required for your bowels). Liquorice tea may also help to get you going (avoid if you have high blood pressure, though).

Still no pleasure?

Do you have irritable bowel syndrome such that your sphincter muscles are in a constant state of contraction, leading to a painful cramping sensation as well? Try high dose Magnesium with B group vitamins, your body's natural muscle relaxants.

TREATMENT FOR CONSTIPATION

Good Quality Probiotics; 2 capsules before breakfast
Dried Figs, Prunes, Apricots
Olive or Flaxseed Oil
Liquorice Tea
Psyllium Husks (2-3 tablespoons as tolerated)
Aloe Vera (Maximum Dose as Directed)
Slippery Elm (Maximum Dose as Directed)
Vitamin C to Bowel Tolerance (until Diarrhoea)

If accompanied by Bowel Spasm:
Magnesium oxide (preferably) (500 mg elemental) plus B Complex

If all else fails, time to make a formal appointment with your doctor.

What about diarrhoea? First of all, pardon the question, are you actually constipated, but with a little fluid flowing around the blockage? You may not be aware of this as it often only shows on an X-ray in the form of faecal impaction, but keep this in mind if the following fails to have effect.

Otherwise, you may have a stomach bug that needs to be eradicated, a food that you should eliminate from your diet, or perhaps a medication that does not agree with you. Still, you should always keep in the back of your mind that any ongoing change of bowel habit is a warning sign, and should not be ignored. Your doctor should always be informed if diarrhoea persists for more than a few days.

This said, you should have already considered a Food Elimination diet with probiotics if you've read this book this far. If you have not undertaken this exercise, read no further. Organise a time to perform this regime now.

So what is left but to detect any irritating bug plaguing your system? Conventional pathology labs can detect most bugs when you send them stool samples. Please note, however, that some bugs are hard to pick up, hence the necessity for three different samples ideally from three different specimens. You will need a doctor's referral and the results should be ready in three days. If these are clear, it may also be important to consider more complicated testing such as CDSAs (Comprehensive Digestive Stool Analyses). Such analyses are available from specialised pathology laboratories (see Appendix). A full analysis entails far more than infective causes.

After which, the use of specifically relevant drug and/ or herbal agents may be needed to eradicate the cause.

Meanwhile, as you wait for either your body (most cases of acute diarrhoea are self healed) or supplementation to kick in, maintain your fluids and electrolytes. Electrolyte ice blocks are effective here and can be purchased from your local chemist. Another option is oat bran, a soluble fibre that may absorb the fluids secreted in your bowel.

And if diarrhoea or constipation continues after these interventions, discuss with your doctor.

ACUTE TREATMENT FOR DIARRHOEA

Maintain Fluids and Electrolytes
Increase Probiotics
Oat Bran

If the condition persists, have a stool analysis performed and treat with appropriate medical or herbal agents as indicated.
e.g Olive Leaf Extract, Artemesia, Oregano Oil, Citrus Seed Extract, Black Walnut etc

So let us return to the beginning. You are what you eat, and you are eating right. You've done your Food Elimination Regime and understand why. What else might be necessary to heal your stomach dysfunction?

Let us follow your food down. First of all there is a simple aid to good digestion. It's as simple as this. Chew. And slosh your food with saliva. This is where digestion begins. Chew well. Put your fork down if you are a compulsive fast eater until every morsel is physically broken down. Meanwhile, enzymes in your saliva get a chance to work. Isn't it obvious? This is why we have teeth. Teeth that, by the way, need to be cleaned regularly. Interestingly, tooth and gum diseases are strongly implicated as factors in cardiovascular disease, so take care of your gums also!

Next, your food reaches your stomach where it is flooded with hydrochloric acid and enzymes to break down the proteins. So here is the next question. Do you have enough acid in your stomach when you eat? Or too much?

Too much or too little hydrochloric acid (HCl) can be the cause of digestive problems, but this really needs to be carefully determined rather than assuming one case or the other, and suffering the side effects of mistreatment.

Unfortunately, this is also an area in which complementary practitioners and medical doctors can be polarised in their opinions, the former tending towards viewing a lack of HCl as the most likely problem, while doctors are more fearful of excess HCl in the stomach. Both alternatives are possible. But getting it wrong has the potential to be dangerous.

For instance, the use of HCl supplements places you at the risk of peptic ulcers, if, in fact, hyperchlorhydria exists. On the other hand, the long-term use of antacids for assumed hyperchlorhydria, particularly if insufficient HCl is being secreted by the stomach, can also lead to complications.

Yes, you can take hydrochloric acid supplements if you are not secreting enough HCl naturally during digestion and you can take antacids (e.g. sodium bicarbonate) if you are secreting too much HCl, but which is relevant to you is the question. We do not want you to be taking antacids if you don't have enough acid in the first place, or taking acid supplements when you are already naturally secreting too much, because both may result in worsening health. This you must leave to a nutritionally orientated doctor or naturopathic practitioner to work on **IF** all else suggested here fails.

It is recommended that you only use HCl support (Betaine Hydrochloride) or antacids (Sodium Bicarbonate) after assessment by a doctor or naturopath who has appropriately assessed your particular circumstances.

There are simpler places to start. Consume a glass of filtered water with one teaspoon of apple cider vinegar, Angosturas bitters or lemon juice (not all together) before your meals. This helps stimulate HCl secretion naturally if required.

You can also take enzymes to help break down your food. Different enzymes work in different areas of your stomach and small intestines, aiding digestion of particular foods such as carbohydrates, proteins (including lactose from milk, which may be helpful if you are intolerant to dairy products) and cellulose, so a broad spectrum enzyme supplement may be helpful. They are good when dining out and allow for spontaneity in your diet when the occasion arises. But remember that digestive enzymes are simply a bandaid and do not help fix the cause of the problem. They only last in the body for several hours, meaning you will need to keep using them before every meal.

TO AID DIGESTION

Digestive Enzymes (Pepsin, Trypsin, Chymotrypsin, Amylase, Lipase, Lactase)

But again, using digestive enzymes would not be our first choice intervention for minor ailments, nor would it be used even when effective for prolonged periods of time (greater than three months). After all, we really do encourage you to use supplements wisely and then wean yourself from them to allow your own body to respond normally once recovered.

So what is our first port of call?

Probiotics.

We have already briefly mentioned probiotics. But what are they? Let's keep it simple. When your digestive tract is in a good state, it is full of billions of foreign bugs known as probiotics, of which there are hundreds of different species. In fact you have more happy little helping bugs in your digestive tract than you do cells in the rest of your body.

There is, in fact, more of you that isn't you than is you if you choose to think about it!

We absolutely need these good bugs. They have a role in helping break down your foods. They also wage a constant battle with bad bugs entering your system to rule their universe, your stomach. Let the bad bugs win and all manner of things run out, so to speak. And not just diarrhoea, many a vitamin and mineral is lost in the bargain.

Unfortunately, we sometimes kill the good bugs and need them to be replaced. How? Poor food choices that feed bad bugs better than the good ones. But worse still, antibiotics. Yes, you might need antibiotics but they do have side effects. They kill all of your bugs, both good and bad. So the good bugs need to be replaced. And that may be all you need to get your gastrointestinal tract back in order, if you're lucky.

What is a good quality probiotic? One that counts its bugs in the billions. And has a wide range of good fellows. Traditionally it has been common to only get three strains of bug or less per capsule—often lactobacillus acidophilus and casei and bifidobacteria bfidium— but as our knowledge progresses, look for multi-strain dosages with different races of good bugs on the market (usually starting with lactobacillus and bifidobacterium, but with different last names, again dosages in the multimillions, billions or more).

START WITH A GOOD PROBIOTIC

Lactobacillus acidophilus	(>2 billion)
Lactobacillus casei	(>1 billion)
Bifidobacterium bifidum	(>500 million)

Other good bugs include Lactobacillus rhamnosus and fermentum, Bifidobacterium breve and longum, but this list will likely grow with future research.

Is this all you need do? Hopefully, but what if you're not so lucky? What else might you need to consider.

At this point we are at the stomach, and we should repeat again what we spoke of in regards to diarrhoea; we need to selectively poison the bad bugs. What to do here? Depends on the bugs you have. And therein lies the problem. Many herbal remedies are known for their antimicrobial activity, but which is the herb for you?

Raw or supplemented garlic, olive leaf extract, goldenseal, barberry bark, oregano oil, wormwood, citrus seed extract, echinacea, Paul D'arco, astragalus, fresh coriander and the list continues. And what each product contains and in what amounts will obviously differ.

Your choice. If probiotics and the Food Elimination Regime haven't worked and you still have diarrhoea, choosing a product will be hit or miss depending upon whether you match a particular supplement to the fungus, bacteria or parasite infiltrating your system. To be more accurate, you may need a stool analysis. Do you want to try a herbal supplement first? The choice is yours, but the obvious solution is to see a practitioner if preliminary self treatment is unsuccessful.

What else might be going on if the bad bugs are winning and your digestion is suffering in turn?

Well, you might have 'leaky gut'. What's that? As simple as it sounds: your gut is leaking. So, what is it leaking? Particles larger than would normally get through the gut wall. Large undigested food fragments, toxins or parasites that would otherwise be weeded out by the physical barrier of a normal gut wall or the effective immune systems found there.

Here are two facts that will probably surprise you.

What provides 70 per cent of your immune system defence?

Your lymph nodes? Your skin? Your liver?

No. Your gut wall. This is where you have the greatest risk of pathogens entering your system. From the food you eat or anything else you might put in your mouth. The reality is, most natural foods are full of toxins before we ever start polluting them. So would you be, if someone was going to eat you! But we neutralise their harmful effects through an effective gut wall immune system. We win the biological and chemical war of survival between a food that doesn't want to be eaten and a gut that wants to eat!

That is, unless we treat our stomachs and intestines badly with poor food choices and toxic assault. In which case, they become leaky and in pour large particles that shouldn't be there. And where do they go? From your bloodstream through your entire system, overburdening the remainder of your body, including your brain. And what happens once these particles reach their unintended destination? The body mounts protective immune system responses leading to inflammatory states where we do not want them. That is, among the functioning cells of our vital health systems. This is why food intolerances can cause so many widespread problems, from headaches and cloudiness to aching arthritic joints.

So if we have treated our gastrointestinal system badly, what do we need to do? Treat it right! Remove the foods that irritate it along with the chemical load we add through non-organic foods, colourings, preservatives and so forth. Give your gut the help of healthy bugs. Soften life in the stomach with some slippery elm or aloe vera. And provide your stomach wall with key nutrients for rebuilding it.

What are they?

Omega-3 fish oils help. As you now know, healthy flexible cell membranes are effectively built from Omega-3 fish oils, and within any gut there is literally kilometres of gut cell membrane. You also need to provide your gut with quality proteins including, most importantly, glucosamine and glutamine, needed to effectively rebuild the gut wall. However, given the widespread effects of leaky gut upon digestion, and the supportive nutrients and amino acids required to rebuild the gut wall, a wider package of nutrients is usually necessary to optimise gut wall repair AND overcome any nutrient deficiencies that have resulted from its recent ineffectiveness.

GUT WALL REPAIR

Omega-3 Fish Oils	EPA/DHA	4 to 9 grams
Glutamine		1000-1500mg
Glucosamine		1500mg

Together with comprehensive multivitamin/ mineral support (preferably in powdered form).
Aloe Vera and Slippery Elm (maximum dosages as recommended).

Finally, to the question of 'detoxification'. While most of what we will write on detoxification is addressed in the following chapter on the liver, it is important to realise that the first organ of detoxification is actually the gut wall. Simply put, it is better that toxins do not get in your system in the first place, rather than needing to be cleaned out of the bloodstream by the liver.

So any program to support the function of the liver equally applies to repairing the gut wall, or, indeed, most digestive system problems. In fact finding solutions to digestive system problems should necessarily precede any consideration of the classic 'liver detoxification'.

After all, if what you put into your digestive system, along with the fact that it is leaking large toxic particles, is not remedied, what is the point of addressing the health of the liver?

Because you are simply going to keep flooding it with new compounds to detoxify anyway.

So always think gut first.

Now let us consider the liver.

3

Demystifying the Liver

Review the following questions to establish whether you have additional reason to consider supporting your liver function.

1. Have you a history of hepatitis, alcohol or recreational drug abuse? Yes / No
2. Are you a smoker? Yes / No
3. Have you been on long-term medication? Yes / No
4. Do you use multiple medications (>than 3)? Yes / No
5. Are you on any high potency medications? Yes / No
6. Have you had recent anaesthetic, chemo or radiotherapy? Yes / No
7. Do you have a history of excess exposure to environmental toxins (Pesticides, Petrochemicals, EMF, Heavy Metals etc)? Yes / No
8. Do you have multiple chemical sensitivities? Yes / No
9. Have you had long-term gastrointestinal problems? Yes / No

Diagnosable diseases specifically involving liver dysfunction include:

✦ Cirrhosis of the Liver, Hepatitis, Fatty Liver Disease
✦ Multiple Chemical Sensitivity Syndrome

Has ever a medical hypothesis received such diverse attention as the subject of liver detoxification? From the 'if in doubt, treat the liver' ethos of traditional naturopaths to the disbelief of conventional medical doctors, the liver is seldom without controversy. It's an amazing organ, able to rejuvenate itself from a slice the size of a coin back to its full might and power, and indeed deserves respect, but can everything said about it be true?

Let us take a simple look at the liver in its role as a detoxifying organ (in fact just one of its many roles) and demystify its function.

First of all, 'detoxifying the liver' should not be seen as a process that only involves the liver. The liver is not one big sponge with the unfortunate plight of absorbing all the toxins you can throw at it, only to be squeezed clean by the act of 'detoxification'. Instead, the liver is an organ that has the role of breaking down toxins as they circulate through the body after being released from the rest of our body's cells. In fact, a 'liver detoxification' should be viewed as a cleansing of the whole body, where each cell is encouraged to release any stored toxin. Remember, every cell in itself acts as a local liver, with its own small-scale detoxifying unit.

Where do the toxins come from? First of all, the liver has always had a role in our lives when it comes to detoxification. When the earth was clean and good and everything was right with the world, the liver was still battling away with natural toxins absorbed from the environment. In fact, all plants have a vast array of toxins amongst the nutrients they supply, as do the animals that eat them and are in turn eaten by us. For each plant and animal in itself evolved natural protection against viruses, bacteria, fungi and indeed other plants and animals. All of which, if consumed, the body must counter if it is to survive.

So we ingested such chemicals and hoped our gut, liver and individual cell detoxification processes got hold of them before they did any harm. And since most of the natural poisons in the environment came via the gastrointestinal tract, and hence were soon after filtered through the liver, our bodies developed an effective process of cleansing.

But things have changed. Not only do we have a vast array of new chemicals to deal with that our bodies have never seen before, but they arrive through many different routes. Through our skin (via soaps, shampoos, lotions, sprayed agents such as fertilisers and herbicides etc), our lungs (fumes from industry, petrochemicals, cigarette smoke) and from unstable dental amalgams (mercury), while far more exotic chemicals pass via the traditional route of our gut.

Here is a list of some of the new chemical threats to our system the previous century has thrown at us:

- Pesticides and herbicides, usually in the form of organophosphates and chlorides.
- An enormous array of chemical formulas found in soaps, shampoos, antiperspirants, detergents, cleansers, aerosols and so forth.
- Food additives and preservatives.
- Prescription medications.
- Out-gassing from carpets along with chemicals emitted from office printers.
- Pool water chlorination.
- Drinking water fluoridation.
- Plastic residues that emit xenoestrogens when left out in the sun, particularly pertinent to drinking water bottles.
- Petrochemical fumes.
- Lead exposure from paints and plumbing in old buildings and atmospheric pollution.
- Mercury from unstable amalgams, cosmetics and as accumulated in large predatory fish (tuna, salmon, shark, swordfish etc).
- Aluminium from cans, cooking pots, antiperspirants, cigarette filters, fabric softeners.
- Cadmium and nickel from cigarette smoking, both active and passive.

So there you have it, in summary a lot more chemicals than the liver is traditionally designed to handle. So when it is argued that the liver's job is to detoxify and therefore it doesn't need any help, you have a simple counterargument.

We suggest that your liver would appreciate help. Not by some magical detoxification diet or list of supplements. No. Simply by limiting your exposure to toxins by using sensible natural alternatives to the long list of chemicals above.

Remember, you will still need to do your research on products; natural does not always mean healthier (and advertising a product as natural does not always mean it is so, therefore learn to read and interpret labels). But you do have a much better chance with a natural product than, for example, a shampoo with a long list of chemicals to its name. There are a whole host of books on this subject, so we will not even try and do the subject justice here. Make it a priority. The first step to a clean system is not to clog it up with chemicals in the first place.

The simplest solutions will begin at home for you may not have the chance to implement change elsewhere. So start by looking at:

- Your foods. Consider organic or homegrown, or at least freshly purchased and local foods.
- Filtering your water.
- Selecting less toxic bathroom products: soaps, shampoos, conditioners, perfumes, antiperspirants, nail polishers, mascara and eye-liners, skin care products.
- Modifying your household cleansers in all their variants: carpet, floor, dishwashing, dishwasher, oven cleaner, window cleaner etc.
- Choosing healthy paints when redecorating. Painting a whole house in non-toxic paints can be cost prohibitive but a room at a time is affordable. Especially important for new babies' rooms. Otherwise, try to have the house painted (or wood stained) when you know you will be away for a few days.
- New carpets. You're in a similar situation when it comes to carpets. These are best allowed to sit before laying in order to out-gas. This may be difficult to do with a new house but easier with new rooms.
- Know what termite treatments have been used in the wood surrounding your house. Do not let your children play on chrome copper arsenic treated playground equipment (often a pine wood with an artificial olive green colour).
- Furthermore, follow the occupational health and safety principles meant to protect you in the workplace and replicate such principles if you do DIY tasks at home.

- Swim in non-chlorinated pools if you have the choice, or at the beach (if not polluted).
- And of course, stop smoking.

Remember, however, that you are not going to be able to live in a bubble. Nor do you want to. Toxins will find a way into your body, they always have, they always will. Particularly vulnerable areas for toxin build-up include your body fat and your brain (a high fat organ), as fat tends to accumulate toxins faster than other tissue. Don't panic, your body is a durable beast and given your willingness to optimise your health, your body will deal with it to the best of its abilities. After which a little added guidance will assist in optimising your health.

So how do we get this toxic build-up out of our bodies?

First of all it is important to highlight that we are only discussing here subtle approaches to chemical build-up that you may be able to implement yourself. There are more complicated medical procedures for removing toxins from the body such as chelation therapy and mercury amalgam removal, but these techniques should only be handled by qualified nutritional and dental specialists trained extensively in these forms of therapy.

After all, to repeat, the toxins are not solely stored in the liver. They are present throughout the body, and to release these toxins safely requires a knowledge of how not only to remove the toxins from the cells in question, but the whole body, without doing harm. Mercury amalgam removal is a good example of this, for such a technique may release more mercury than the filling was leaching in the first place if performed incorrectly!

You have already had an insight into detoxification. We have already talked about natural cellular detoxification processes when we discussed cellular health. Remember the four powerful sounding enzymes present in our cells; superoxide dismutase, glutathione perioxidase, perioxinitrite and metallothionein. To keep it simple, these compounds need the help of minerals (zinc, copper, selenium, magnesium) to keep the process going along with essential amino acids (e.g. glutamine, glutathione, cysteine, methionine etc).

Exercise, massage and steam baths may also help to mobilise toxins through perspiration, as may weight loss, due to the break down of adipose tissue where toxins are preferentially stored. Here's a treat; lie in a hot bath filled with half a cup of Epsom salts, half a cup of apple cider vinegar and a few drops of lavender oil for a wonderful gentle detoxification. Try this for a few days in a row for maximum benefit.

Any toxin released from the cells that has not been neutralised eventually reaches the liver.

So what happens once toxins get here?

Lets look at the 'simple' science of the liver's role of detoxification rather than the vast array of non-scientific myth.

The liver proceeds through a two-step process of detoxification for any toxin. The first step is undertaken for all toxins, regardless of their nature. It is called **Phase 1 Detoxification**. This phase is like a general purpose rubbish collection in preparation for selective processing. A toxin entering the liver is transformed into an intermediate molecule. That is, a molecule that is only halfway through the detoxification process. The body creates intermediate molecules to make the toxin amenable to the toxin specific processes of Phase 2. After Phase 1 it is important to note that the intermediate molecule remains toxic. Only after both phases are complete is a toxin safe to the body.

Therefore whether Phase 1 is under or overactive, it can cause a problem. If Phase 1 is overactive, too many toxic intermediate molecules result that are unable to be processed quickly enough through Phase 2 Detoxification. This can often be the case after excessive use of alcohol, nicotine, stress, prescription drug use including steroids, or excess exposure to environmental toxins.

This results in the need for added Antioxidant Nutrients (see Cellular Health) due to increased free radical exposure. Grapefruit (in whole or extract form) and the herb, St Mary's Thistle, also aid this situation, by down regulating over-reactive Phase 1 Liver Detoxification.

On the other hand, if Phase 1 is underactive, often due to the overuse of another list of prescription drugs such as benzodiazepines (valium), then the liver is slow in passing toxins on to the next phase of processing, hence not doing its job adequately. Thus the potential need for supplements that support this process; the compound glutathione or the amino acids that help to create it; glycine, glutamine and cysteine (all found in quality protein sources), with the assistance of Methionine and N-acetyl cysteine, the B group vitamins, Magnesium, Selenium and Zinc (you may remember these as the nutrients supporting enzyme detoxification in the cells, see Cellular Health).

Are you starting to get the idea that the nutritional science behind liver detoxification is not that simple? Sorry, some body processes just can't be simplified, even if it is the one process that everyone wants to simplify!

And **Phase 2 Detoxification** doesn't get any simpler. As previously mentioned, Phase 2 consists of four separate pathways depending on the toxin in question, known as Glutathionation, Sulphation, Glucuronidation and Glycination. And each of the pathways requires different considerations.

Glutathionation is responsible for dealing with toxins such as pesticides, paracetamol, toxic metals, alcohol and petrol products. Similar nutrients as for Phase 1 detoxification are required. The cruciferous vegetables such as broccoli and cauliflower also support this pathway.

Sulphation works upon breaking down the steroid hormones (sex hormones and DHEA), histamine, noradrenaline and adrenaline. It requires sulphur rich amino acids to be functional; Taurine, Cysteine, Methionine and the trace mineral, Molybdenum. Which are also available from sulphur rich foods such as eggs, nuts, broccoli, brussels sprouts, artichoke, seeds, cabbage, cauliflower and turnip.

Glucuronidation also helps to detoxify sex hormones, paracetamol, valium and benzodiazepines. It requires Magnesium, Zinc, Essential Fatty Acids and Vitamin B Complex. The herb turmeric (curcumin) is also helpful here.

Glycination detoxifies salicylic acid (aspirin). Glycine, Vitamin B6 and Magnesium help this path proceed. Since this path is detoxifying salicylic acid, a reduction in the use of salicylates, antihistamines and nasal decongestants as found in many over-the-counter medications is also recommended if this path is underactive.

Complicated? Of course, there are some reasons why medical professionals and naturopaths go to universities and health schools. Is the above going to help you work out a protocol for your own liver detoxification?

Probably not. Not specifically anyway. After all, how are you going to know whether your Phase 1 is up, down or perfect, and whether or not your Glucuronidation, Glycation, Sulphation, Glycination and the whole complicated process of your Phase 2 balance is in order?

How does your doctor know? Well, actually, standard medical trained doctors rarely investigate your liver detoxification profiles to this extent. Yes, they do liver tests called 'Liver Function Tests' or LFT's, but LFT's do not measure exactly what the liver is doing, rather they measure how much of it is damaged. To know how effectively your liver is detoxifying, you need a Functional Liver Detoxification Profile. Many doctors will not necessarily know what this is but it can be accessed through a nutritionally orientated doctor, and in many instances, a naturopath or nutritionist (see Appendix).

So if you suspect you have a less than perfect liver, perhaps due to the use of multiple medications, alcohol, or exposure to environmental toxins, or you have symptoms such as multiple chemical sensitivities, hormonal problems that are resistant to treatment, intolerances to food, chronic fatigue, headaches or migraine, any number of treatment resistant gastrointestinal symptoms or widespread muscle aches and pains that have been resistant to first line treatment, it may be time to seek out a medical professional who can order more extensive tests than simple LFT's, in order to more accurately devise a treatment plan for effectively improving your liver function.

What if you want to simply enhance your liver function, without the need for such an analysis?

Well there are simple keys within the discussion so far that are easy to follow, without the need for supplements. These include:

- Limit your exposure to as many environmental toxins as listed above as possible.
- Drink lots of water. The end products of liver detoxification are near water soluble particles that are excreted through bile or urine, therefore high fluid intake is necessary for toxin excretion.
- Stop drinking alcohol and coffee and quit smoking.
- Do not take any recreational or over-the-counter drugs.
- If possible, but only after discussion with your doctor, limit your use of prescription drugs.

- Maintain your protein intake at one to two meals per day using the hand measure. Consume high quality, low fat, organic meats or eggs (unless you have high cholesterol) in order to consume the essential amino acids required for liver detoxification. Small fresh fish are preferable; large predatory fish are not.
- Perform the Food Elimination Regime outlined in Section 3, Chapter 8. This is a good time to investigate your Food Intolerances.
- Grapefruit is generally an excellent food, but this assumes you do not have a low Phase 1. If you eat grapefruit and your symptoms worsen, stop. Always check with your pharmacist or doctor if grapefruit interacts with any prescription medication you are taking.
- Consume plenty of fruit and vegetables, especially from the sulphur containing vegetables (broccoli, cauliflower, brussel sprouts) listed above as aiding Sulphation. Doubly effective are the cruciferous vegetables that aid Glutathionation.
- Use natural herbs to flavour your food including turmeric, which aids Glucuronidation.
- A mix of fresh nuts and seeds (raw, unsalted) will help provide a broad base of vitamins and minerals.
- Get plenty of fresh air, exercise, mineral baths, and if available, massages and steam baths (as long as adequately hydrated).
- Relax and enjoy non-stressful living including pleasure activities and learning to utilise positive emotions.
- Remember that early 'Liver Detoxification' is often associated with a few days of discomfort as the toxins are initially released into your system.

And if you want to supplement?

Well, most of what the liver needs is actually what the entire body needs, because each and every single cell needs to individually perform detoxification. You can look at Cellular Health, therefore, and revise by considering the use of:

LIVER DETOXIFICATION (see also 'Cellular Health')

Essential Fatty Acids
Omega-3 Fish Oil   4-9g
Antioxidants
B Complex
Magnesium (elemental)   500mg

And additional consideration may be given to a three-month regime of:

St Mary's Thistle   Up to 10-20g
Globe Artichoke Leaf   500mg
Taurine   500mg
Glycine   500mg bedtime

Additional Support for Detoxifying Enzymes as per Practitioner (See Chapter 1 of this section, 'Cellular Health')

A further note should be added for people who have difficulty digesting fatty foods. This may be caused by a poorly functioning gall bladder. The role of the gall bladder is to secrete enzymes within bile that are responsible for fat absorption in the intestine. In turn, this is also related to the inability of the liver to clear fats from itself. Remembering that the role of the liver is to detoxify fat soluble toxins so that they can be excreted through the gut (as well as urine), the gall-bladder is therefore also important in liver detoxification.

Again, lifestyle changes should be your first line of action including:

+ Following the Healthy Eating Plan to slowly lose weight.
+ Lowering your cholesterol using additional supplementation (as found under Cardiovascular Health). This particularly should include the use of Lecithin Granules, which contain the vital nutrients Inositol and Choline that aid bile salt formation. Taurine may be used as an additional aid.
+ Digestive Enzymes may be used during an interim period to aid digestion.

- Drinking Dandelion Tea is thought to aid the gall bladder as well as the liver.

Note again, vigorous supplementation or medication is an adjunct, not necessarily a first course approach unless symptoms cannot be eradicated with simple lifestyle measures.

So what, in summary, do we have to say about Liver Detoxification?

On the one hand there is a science to understanding nutritional approaches to the liver (as with every organ), so the mainstream view that there is no merit in treating the liver is unacceptable. It is more than a simple science though, often requiring laboratory testing to identify any specific requirements that need to be addressed, and this should therefore be respected.

So why not try respecting your liver for a time by using the simple lifestyle measures we have suggested (with or without supplementation), whether or not you wish to call it simple healthy living, or 'Liver Detoxification'.

Now here's a better thought, why don't you live this way all the time? Follow the simple Healthy Eating Plan in this book, perhaps after an initial 'Liver Detoxification' adjustment as above. Limit your exposure to toxins. Enjoy life.

Remove negative emotional patterns from your behaviours. Live with Passion.

And simply call it:

Life detoxification!

Now that can't be controversial now, can it?

4

Cardiovascular Health

You should carefully consider your cardiac health if one or more of the following are applicable to you:

You have been told that you have high cholesterol by your doctor	Yes / No
There is a family history of heart disease or stroke	Yes / No
You are diabetic	Yes / No
You are a smoker	Yes / No
You are overweight	Yes / No
You have high blood pressure	Yes / No
You are over 40 and have not regularly exercised	Yes / No
You suffer from anxiety or depression	Yes / No

You should see your doctor if you experience any unexplainable chest, abdomen, jaw or upper limb tightness or pain, get short of breath on minimal exertion, wake up at night short of breath, have a recent need to sleep on more than one pillow or have swelling in both ankles.

Diagnosable diseases specifically involving cardiovascular health include:

- ✦ Angina, Heart Attack, Heart Failure
- ✦ Cerebrovascular Accidents (Stroke)
- ✦ Blood Pressure, Peripheral Vascular Disease, Anaemia, Clotting Disorders.

Cardiovascular health can be broken down into a few major focuses.

The most important thing for you to know about the health of your heart is that a lot of it is basically up to you. The eight most commonly cited risk factors for cardiovascular disease in general are high cholesterol, high homocysteine levels, high blood pressure, smoking, diabetes (often as a disease progression from Insulin Resistance), obesity, family history and, a recent addition to the list, depression.

Yes, there are genetic factors, but as has been clearly demonstrated with breast cancer genes, despite a large percentage of individuals inheriting the specific genes, not all of these people actually get breast cancer. The same is true for heart disease. Don't panic if you have a family history of heart disease. But be wise with your lifestyle choices to minimise your future risk. What is true of breast cancer and heart disease applies to almost all genetic inheritances.

Even though you may be genetically predisposed, you may never actually develop the disease if you live according to healthy life principles.

We certainly do not yet understand all there is to know regarding genetic expression, but there is a very large component that relies on the choices you make in life. Such choices as your diet, your exercise, your lifestyle habits, your stress and your happiness. So, what's new? Again and again, you can see the same themes rearing their common little heads.

Let us look at modifying the cardiac risk factors you can address.

Cholesterol

For many decades, elevated cholesterol has been known to be a significant risk factor for both cardiovascular disease, including atherosclerosis and heart attacks, and cerebrovascular disease, including strokes. This is certainly an extremely important risk factor, as statistics speak for themselves. Like everything in life, there are those individuals who do not suffer with any complications from high cholesterol. This is most definitely the exception to the rule. Cardiovascular disease has a horrible morbidity, as well as mortality rate, which means a very poor quality of life whichever way you look at it. No-one wants this if they can do something to avoid it. And you can.

These days, most people don't gorge themselves on fatty meats, deep-fried foods and rich creamy sauces every day. Not, at least, after they have been told their cholesterol has gone through the roof (given that they are actually concerned about their health). In fact, in our experience …

It's actually the foods people are not eating, rather than those they are eating, that actually constitute the problem.

Simply put, the main food that is not consumed in great enough quantities is fish. Authorities actually recommend at least three servings of fish per week to obtain the right amount of essential fatty acids to maintain optimal cardio-vascular health. The fish that contain the highest amount of good omega-3 essential fatty acids are oily fish such as sardines, herring, mackeral, trevally, salmon and tuna. However, here it needs to be reiterated that large individual fish such as salmon and tuna (also swordfish and shark) are also unfortunately the very same fish that contain the highest amounts of heavy metals such as mercury and contaminants such as dioxins and PCBs. In fact, a recent medical study stated that more than two-three serves of large fish per week may actually raise an individuals dioxin and PCB levels to toxic levels.

This dilemma is only going to get worse. Environmental medicine doctors are only too aware of the widespread toxic effects of mercury and other heavy metals on the health of individuals and, even more significantly, their offspring. So what is the solution? Seek out fresh fish that have been caught in uncontaminated waters (but where are they and how do you know where your fish has come from?).

Or limit your large individual fish intake (steaks and fillets), choose limited smaller fish sources (canned fish are supposedly younger fish who have not yet accumulated high mercury levels through predation), and supplement with quality fish oils that have been screened for heavy metals and other pollutants such as dioxins and PCBs.

So, back to cholesterol. An excess of eggs in the diet may certainly raise some people's cholesterol, but this is a particular sub-group of responders (often Diabetic) and not the majority of people. The only way to see if eggs affect you, however, is to have your own cholesterol checked at three-monthly intervals after an appropriate change in diet. Lots of full-cream dairy products and excess red meat may also raise one's levels. If you are a person with high cholesterol worsened by egg intake, decreasing consumption of these would be the next step after increasing your essential fatty acid intake through healthy fish or nutritional supplementation.

Which brings us to another important point. The ratio of your good cholesterol (HDL) compared to your bad cholesterol (LDL) is the most significant factor of all, not necessarily your overall cholesterol level. If your total cholesterol is high but the majority is derived from HDL, then it is unlikely you actually have a problem. In most Australian pathology labs, the upper limit of LDL is approximately 3.5. If your LDL is above this level, generally you would benefit from some intervention.

There are several different natural regimes that may help to lower LDL cholesterol. In our clinical experience, the regime below followed for three months, combined with a Healthy Eating Plan and moderate exercise, works for the vast majority of people. We find that those individuals who may not respond (<5 per cent in our experience) actually have very strong hereditary factors. Even if this is you, we believe it's still worth a try.

CHOLESTEROL LOWERING REGIME

EPA/DHA fish oils	4g
Vitamin C	3g
Garlic	3g
Psyllium husks	1-2 tbsp
Lecithin granules	1-2 tbsp

It is important to note that the husks of psyllium must be used as the larger surface area is needed to attach to the LDL cholesterol so that it will pass out through your faeces. As we say to all our patients, it doesn't matter how you consume it, whether it's in divided doses three times a day, in yoghurt or cereal, sprinkled on broccoli or in juice, just stick to the same amount for the full three months so that you can determine what amount is actually necessary to maintain optimal levels.

Three more points need to be emphasised in this section. As with all illnesses, sometimes pharmaceutical medications are indeed necessary in treating cholesterol. Many cholesterol lowering medications, primarily the 'statins', as they are known, also lower other levels of important nutrients in the body, like CoQ10. This nutrient is also known as Ubiquitone, because its effects are ubiquitous around the entire body.

In this section, it is vital to mention that adequate levels of CoQ10 are as important as appropriate levels of cholesterol to our cardiovascular health. Coenzyme Q10 has been shown to increase the strength of our heart muscle and acts as an antioxidant, preventing cholesterol from developing into atherosclerotic plaque. Coenzyme Q10 is also needed for energy production in combination with Vitamins B1, B2, B3, B6 and Magnesium and therefore can be helpful in the treatment of fatigue.

HEART HEALTH, PARTICULARLY IF ON A STATIN DRUG

Co-Enzyme Q10	100–200mg
Magnesium (elemental)	500mg
B Complex	
Zinc	15mg
Vitamin E	200IU
Taurine	1000mg

Which brings us to our second point of significance. Cholesterol of itself must oxidise or become inflamed before it transforms into atherosclerotic plaque. Thus it is argued by some that cholesterol levels may not be of major significance **IF** a person has adequate antioxidant levels to protect against free radicals **AND/OR** does not have a pro-inflammatory systemic environment. As mentioned previously, one other factor contributing to cardiac disease is now known to be the presence of peri-dental infections, so brush your teeth!

Therefore further protection against cardiac disease can be achieved by the use of **Broadbased Antioxidant Nutrients** (see 'Cellular Health', Chapter 1 of this section), the avoidance of accumulated toxins through sensible environment choices (including not smoking) and a down-regulation of the immune system towards a less inflammatory state (see Chapter 10, 'Creating a Healthy Immune System').

It should also be noted that there are a multiple of studies demonstrating that Vitamin B3 can work synergistically with CoQ10 +/- statin drugs to lower LDL and raise HDL levels of cholesterol.

INVESTIGATING YOUR PERSONAL SUPPLEMENT NEEDS

ADDITIONAL CHOLESTEROL PROTECTION

Broadbased Antioxidant Supplement
(see 'Cellular Health', Chapter 1 of this section)
Vitamin B3 (niacinamide)—under practitioner supervison

The final point is that levels of cholesterol should be within range, which means neither too high **NOR** too low. For it is from cholesterol that our sex hormones, our adrenal hormones, our vital-for-life hormones, are derived. You should therefore read the chapter on 'Hormone Health' to educate yourself on how incredibly important a role cholesterol plays in the functioning of your entire body. You can't do without it, so do not become obsessed with it and drive it lower that it needs to go.

Homocysteine Levels

A fasting homocysteine level is another test that may be checked if you have a strong family history of cardiovascular disease, learning difficulties, recurrent miscarriages, elevated cholesterol, a lowered Vitamin B12 level, coeliac disease, inflammatory bowel disease or are vegetarian.

Homocysteine is an amino acid derived protein important in too many enzymatic reactions to mention here, except to say that it may be just as important as high cholesterol in determining your cardiovascular health. Unfortunately, when nutrient intake or genetic factors lead to your homocysteine levels being out of balance, you are at risk of a variety of diseases including cardiovascular disease.

Vitamin B12, Vitamin B6 and folic acid are all essential to keep homocysteine levels acceptable. The contingent nutrient, SAMe (S-adenyl-methionine) is also intricately connected in the methylation pathway.

HEALTHY HOMOCYSTEINE LEVELS (THREE-MONTH REGIME)

Vitamin B12	400–1000 ug
Vitamin B6	50–200mg
Folate	400–1000ug
B Complex	
Plus/ minus	
Betaine Hydrochloride	500mg (if not hyperchlorhydric)
SAMe	200mg

Start with low doses for three months, however higher doses may be required if your homocysteine levels are significantly raised, to lower them below 10.

Hypertension

Hypertension or high blood pressure is so incredibly common in today's society that we almost take it for granted. It is important to know that 95 per cent of hypertension is termed 'idiopathic', meaning 'with no known cause'. In contrast, only 5 per cent can be attributable to known causes, such as kidney disease and the like.

Whatever the cause, the possible consequences of hypertension such as strokes, heart attacks and ruptured aneurysms are too important to ignore. High blood pressure must be brought to an acceptable level quickly and this, without doubt, involves the use of pharmaceutical medications. Other complementary approaches may be attempted simultaneously but they will take time to work. And with high blood pressure, time is of the essence. You may be preventing a literal time bomb from going off inside your head and heart. By all means, take high blood pressure seriously.

On a lighter note, it is interesting that the word hypertension is derived from hyper (meaning an excess of) and tension; need we say more? Suffice it to say that there have been multiple studies demonstrating that relaxation improves high blood pressure (in the form of transcendental meditation, mindfulness meditation and yoga, for example). More recently, there have been studies showing how happiness or depression levels are directly linked to your predisposition to developing heart disease.

In fact, it has now been shown that your level of happiness is just as important a risk factor for cardiovascular disease as your direct family history.

We must not forget that weight loss through an appropriate Healthy Eating Plan (high fruit and vegetables, low fats, low fat dairy products) and moderate exercise can achieve wonders. In fact, the 'green prescription' which involves simply a modification of lifestyle factors and choices, is the primary recommendation from most medical doctors these days to prevent high blood pressure.

It is always important to consider the influence hormones may have on blood pressure. In particular, some perimenopausal women experience a rise in blood pressure for no apparent reason. This may be a symptom of hormone imbalance (for example, progesterone deficiency) as much as erratic moods and vagueness.

Nutritionally speaking, there are many varied herbs and nutrients that have been shown to lower blood pressure. In our clinical experience, however, we find hypertension and its appropriate treatment is different for each individual. Unlike our cholesterol regime, there is no definitive answer. Unfortunately, what works for some does not necessarily work for others.

Nutrients worth trying include Omega-3 fish oils, potassium rich foods (fruit and vegetables), magnesium, Vitamin C, Co-Enzyme Q10 and Taurine, although as mentioned, results will vary, as there appears to be a number of sub-groups for people who experience hypertension. There are also various herbs that can have an effect on the lowering of blood pressure but, once again, these are best decided on by an experienced practitioner. A recent supplement on the market, bonito peptides, derived from the bonito tuna fish, is also showing promise, but you'll need to ask a nutritionally orientated practitioner further advice about this.

The key, as usual, would appear to be an integrated approach. Healthy eating, exercise, stress reduction, emotional management, and as an adjunct, nutritional supplementation and/or prescription medication may all be necessary to get high blood pressure under control.

HIGH BLOOD PRESSURE TREATMENT OPTIONS

High fruit and vegetable intake (*as per Healthy Eating Plan*)
Increase potassium rich foods
Lower salt intake (Reduction in canned/processed foods)
Omega-3 fish oils   EPA/DHA   4–6g
Magnesium (elemental)   500mg
B Complex
Vitamin C   3g
Co-Enzyme Q10   100–200mg
Taurine   500mg

Anaemia

A short note on blood. Anaemia is a relatively common occurrence particularly in the elderly, menstruating women and people who have recently undergone surgery. Another group are vegetarians, since the lack of animal protein in the diet also means a lack of iron. Yes, there is iron in vegetarian sourced foods, but unfortunately it is bound by the presence of phytates, which means much of it is flushed directly through your system without being absorbed. This is one area where vegetarianism is not ideal.

The differentiation between animal sourced iron and non-animal sourced iron is categorised by the terms haem and non-haem iron. You need a haem form of iron to be appropriately absorbed as non-haem irons (from vegetable sources) are far less effectively digested. One suggested approach to absorbing non-haem iron sources is to consume iron rich vegetable matter or green drinks (e.g. Spirulina) with Vitamin C, but this is at best a questionable approach.

This is why green juices are not that effective in increasing iron levels despite the claims, while two serves or more of red meat per week will help to raise iron levels. However, this is still a very slow process. For quicker results, choose an iron supplement, preferably with folate. But realise the digestive tract can only consume small quantities of iron at a time, so that the megadose shots in prescription style supplements (up to 100mg at a time) do not necessarily equate to rapid iron increases. They do, however, risk constipating you and turning your faeces various shades of black!

ANAEMIA

Iron (elemental)	35–50mg
Folate	500ug

One note of caution. One in 400 people have haemochromatosis, a disorder of iron excess. In this case, you should not take iron supplements as it will subsequently risk iron accumulating in the body with long-term negative effects. Excess intake of iron can also be pro-inflammatory and lower the function of the immune system. Therefore, you should seek advice from your doctor regarding balanced iron levels if you have inflammatory or infective conditions. Please note that even though you may not be anaemic (haemoglobin >110) you may still be iron deficient. As this is extremely common, it is always advisable to check your ferritin levels. The normal range of ferritin is usually considered to be 15–300; however, nutritionally orientated doctors consider a midrange of ferritin acceptable. This means a lower limit of 55 with an ideal level of 100 or above.

If you are a person who bruises frequently you may lack Vitamin K (from leafy green vegetables), Vitamin C or the Bioflavonoid group, all of which assist in clotting. However this is another area where you need to be careful, particularly if you are on medications such as Warfarin. If not on medication you should be OK to supplement, assuming you have discussed with your doctor any of the reasons that may exist for slow clotting, but if on medication you will need to heed your doctor's or pharmacist's advice on whether supplementation is appropriate for you (in the case of Warfarin, Vitamin K supplementation definitely is not!).

EXCESS BRUISING

Vitamin K	2–5ug
Vitamin C with Bioflavonoids	3 grams

On the other hand, do you have a concern about clotting? Perhaps you have a family history of heart disease, embolic stroke or peripheral vascular disease, or you simply do not want the risk of deep vein thrombosis from a long haul flight. Assuming you are not on medication (talk to your doctor first if you are), you could try the blood thinning agents garlic, ginger or gingko biloba. In some individuals, horse chestnut may also assist with peripheral circulation and varicose veins.

5

Respiratory and Airways Health

The following advice in this chapter is pertinent if:

You have a history of smoking	**Yes / No**
You suffer from breathing difficulties	**Yes / No**
Concerns regarding your breathing make you anxious	**Yes / No**
You frequently cough up phlegm	**Yes / No**
You have a frequent dry cough	**Yes / No**
You regularly experience lung, throat or sinus infections	**Yes / No**

Diagnosable diseases specifically involving the respiratory system include:

- ✦ Emphysema, Bronchitis, Bronchiectasis
- ✦ Asthma, Hay Fever, Sinusitis

Go without food for several days to weeks and your health is at critical risk.

Go without water for several hours to days and your life quickly deteriorates.

Go without air in your lungs for several minutes ... DEAD!

Now, that's simple!

Given this, your lungs, in most instances, are very resilient organs. A normal healthy set of lungs will last you a lifetime, and only deteriorate at a slow enough pace to match the general decline in your activity levels.

Unless, that is, you choose to poison them!

And even when you poison them with nicotine, cadmium, aluminium, nickel and a whole host of nasties in both cigarette and filter, your lungs usually struggle along for a good few decades before the rot sets in. That's the long-suffering lungs' problem, they suffer abuse readily but only deteriorate slowly. They do not suddenly attack you with a stroke or heart attack. And so they get taken for granted until extreme breathlessness sets in. And by then it is too late.

For once your lung has a problem severe enough for you to you notice it, there is often little you can do short of drastic measures. You generally either have lung cancer or emphysema, both of which are serious diseases rather than dysfunctions and beyond the scope of this book to discuss.

So you should realise that ...

Far more than for most of your body's systems and organs, the lungs need to be acknowledged before you are given any warning sign that they are in trouble. And 99 per cent of the time, that acknowledgement comes down to one simple message, and one simple choice.

Don't pollute your lungs ...

QUIT SMOKING!

Of course there are other potential pollutants to be aware of that may also cause a decline in your lungs. In most instances, this comes down to being aware of the pollutants that are present predominantly in your work environment (asbestos, aerosols, detergents, farming agents such as fertilisers and herbicides, paint solvents, petrol, diesel and chemical fumes involved in manufacturing) but also during DIY tasks (use industrial masks), hobbies, and bird keeping (especially pigeons).

But ultimately, the most common risk to your lungs is simple. Smoking. You know it. The cigarette packet tells you the fact of the matter. So all we can say is, however you can do it, minimise or quit smoking. And not only for yourself. For the people who are passively smoking in your fumes around you, particularly young infants and babies at risk of developing asthma, or worse still, Sudden Infant Death Syndrome.

Giving up smoking may not be easy. It is both a physical and emotional addiction. In fact it is an amazing means of medicating (blunting) against both the 'ups' (nervousness, anxiety) and 'downs' (poor concentration, depression) of negative emotions. But your health in later life depends on it. The occasional lucky centurion is a smoker as typified by comedian George Burns, and our humour-filled grandfather, George Bryson, but these are the exceptions, and they are far from the rule. They won the lucky genetic lottery. Most don't!

And smoking won't just attack your lungs either. Few if any forms of cancer are immune from the negative influences of smoking. Your gastrointestinal system is affected by smoking. Your heart health is at risk from smoking. Your liver and every other cell in your body needs to work hard at clearing up the toxins of smoking. Your blood vessels are susceptible to the impact of smoking, particularly if diabetic. Which means every small ending of the arteries in your toes, fingers, eyes, kidneys, but also your brain, will decline under the influence of smoking.

So find whatever resources you can to aid in quitting smoking. And you will need help. Long-term success for quitting smoking runs at only around one in four smokers, even when supported by clinics, so it is no easy task. The use of the supplements Tryptophan, Tyrosine and other precursors to Dopamine, details of which can be found in 'Neurotransmitter Health' (Chapter 8 of this section), may assist with anxiety and cravings. B Complex and magnesium can help counter the stressful effects of withdrawal. A broadbased antioxidant and immune system support (to counter the long-term effects of smoking) may help too, but ultimately psychological counselling and medication may also be needed by some.

Note that eventually nicotine gum and patches also need to be overcome, as they simply change the mode of nicotine entry into the body (saving the lungs in preference to harming elsewhere).

Good luck! We wish you the very best! The battle may not be easy, but the health rewards are definitely worth it.

QUIT SMOKING SUPPLEMENT SUPPORT

Tryptophan or tyrosine (see *'Neurotransmitter Health'*, Chapter 8 of this section)
Magnesium (elemental)   500mg
B Complex
Broad based antioxidant (see *'Cellular Health'*, Chapter 1 of this section)

Plus Immune System Support
(see *'Creating a Healthy Immune System'*, Chapter 10 of this section)

Airways

The airways of your body require special consideration. These not only include your trachea and the bronchi leading to your lungs, but also the nasal cavity and air-containing sinuses within your skull.

Asthma is a disease of the respiratory tract. Think of your upper airway as a hollow tube whose width and hence air carrying capacity is determined by two components. On the inner layer is your mucosal tissue, not dissimilar to the lining of your mouth. Within it are immune system cells that, if they become hypersensitive, cause swelling of the mucosa and the secretion of phlegm, hence resulting in a narrowing of your airways.

The outer perimeter of your airways is made up of circular muscles that, if they contract, also narrow the airways. This contraction will again occur under the influence of the immune system if the latter perceives a stimulus in the environment that it considers to be unhealthy. The immune system of an asthmatic considers certain normal environmental stimuli as abnormal, hence triggering inappropriate swelling and muscle contractions that in turn cause inappropriate narrowing of the airways.

The result: shortness of breath, difficulty performing activities, coughing, phlegm and so forth. How do we address this response?

1. Minimise the hyper-responsiveness of the immune system by minimising triggers.
2. Minimise smooth muscle contraction.
3. Reduce the swelling that results from immune system hyperactivity.

There are, of course, medical approaches based on the above, but what are the complementary approaches that may aid with asthma?

1. Where possible, the first course of action is environmental change. Establish your triggers and minimise them where possible.
    (i) Airborne irritants may include dust mites, cats, dogs, food vapours (even if not digested), heating gases, paints and solvents, petrochemicals, vacuum cleaner dusts, moulds and, obviously, cigarette smoke. Each of these triggers can be minimised with due care, so investigate your particular trigger through appropriate asthma directed literature.
    (ii) Cow's milk is a common food intolerance and may be a trigger for both asthma and sinusitis. But a variety of foods may be implicated including a variety of fruit and vegetables with high salicylate load and foods dried with sulphur agents. So to find this out, a Food Elimination Regime is in order, starting with a course of probiotics.
    (iii) Salicylate medication may also affect some asthmatics.
    (iv) Exercise may trigger some asthmatics, although this does not imply exercise should be stopped, rather performed with due care e.g. if required, always have your bronchodilator medication (such as Ventolin) available. Exercise induced asthmatics are a subgroup which may respond to Vitamin C, three grams daily.

2. Try a B complex with high dose magnesium as a natural muscle relaxant for airways constriction, not unlike the recommendations for cramp or muscle spasm.
3. After which, address balancing the immune system with EPA/ DHA fish oils, Vitamin C, garlic, zinc, and antioxidants. See 'Creating a

Healthy Immune System' (Chapter 10 of this section) for more guidance.

4. There is evidence to support Buteyko Breathing for asthma sufferers, although clinical applications of this technique are far more widespread. There are also many herbal and homeopathic remedies that may help reduce lung congestion and improve airway health, but we would recommend you seek advice from a complementary health practitioner before using these.

Similar approaches can be taken for hay fever and sinusitis, since they are also hyper-reactivity disorders of the immune system. The main difference, as compared to the treatment of asthma, is that there is no smooth muscle involvement in the nasal cavity and sinuses, therefore specific magnesium and B Complex supplementation is not necessary.

ASTHMA, HAY FEVER, SINUSITIS

Identify and Mminimise your personal triggers
Food Elimination Regime
Broad based antioxidant support (see 'Cellular Health', Chapter 1 of this section)
Immune System Support (see 'Creating a Healthy Immune System', Chapter 10 of this section)

Specifically for asthma
Magnesium (elemental)   500mg
B Complex
Vitamin C (if exercise induced)   3g

6

Insulin Resistance, Diabetes and Weight Loss

You should consider Insulin Resistance a concern if you experience any of the following on a regular basis:

Anxiety, palpitations, fatigue, sleepiness, poor concentration, dizziness, yawning, mild headache, restlessness if a meal is delayed.	Yes / No
If when experiencing any of the above feelings, a high carbohydrate meal relieves your symptoms	Yes / No
You feel the need to eat again 2-3 hours after a high carbohydrate meal.	Yes / No
You eat in response to emotions	Yes / No
You crave high carbohydrate foods	Yes / No
You are overweight	Yes / No
You have Polycystic Ovarian Syndrome	Yes / No

You should be reviewed by your doctor to establish your risk of diabetes if:

You are overweight, over 40 or have a family history of Diabetes	Yes / No
You have an increased frequency of urination, particularly at night	Yes / No
Have unexplained pins and needles in fingers or toes	Yes / No
You are frequently hungry or thirsty without explanation	Yes / No
You are experiencing unexplained dizzy spells	Yes / No

Diagnosable diseases specifically involving insulin resistance include:

- Diabetes
- Obesity
- Cardiovascular Disease including High Blood Pressure
- Polycystic Ovary Disease
- Depression, Anxiety.

Insulin is a very powerful hormone, its primary action being to regulate our blood sugar levels. For a variety of reasons, not all of which are yet completely understood, the pancreas can stop producing insulin (usually in childhood) and the disease Insulin Dependent Diabetes Mellitus subsequently develops. These people rely on injecting themselves with insulin on a daily basis in order to stop themselves developing ongoing hyperglycaemia, coma and eventually death.

The most common type of diabetes, Non-Insulin Dependent Diabetes Mellitus, is, in contrast, a disease that we ultimately should have control over.

The developed nations of the world are currently undergoing an epidemic of this particular type of Diabetes Mellitus. Childhood and adult obesity, insulin resistance, impaired glycemic control, diabetes mellitus: these are all on the same continuum of disease.

Insulin resistance, put simply, is basically the body becoming resistant to the effects of insulin. The role of insulin is to act as the key that opens the lock that allows glucose (energy) into your cells. For a variety of reasons (including, most importantly, a high carbohydrate diet combined with a lack of exercise), the receptors in cell membranes become less and less effective in recognising this hormone and therefore the pancreas produces more and more insulin in an attempt to maintain appropriate blood sugar levels. One area where these receptor locks tend to keep working is in the body fat tissues in the waist region. As a consequence, people with insulin resistance often experience selective waist weight gain, from an oversupply of sugar. Insulin is also labelled an anabolic (or building) hormone, leading to weight gain, as opposed to a catabolic (or breaking down hormone), which would contribute to weight loss.

Eventually, the pancreas is unable to supply enough insulin to maintain stable blood sugar levels and blood sugar levels begin to rise above normal. At this stage you have reached a state in which you may be diagnosed as having Non Insulin Dependent Diabetes Mellitus. Ignore this and the overworking pancreas starts to falter, unable to keep working at the intense pace it has been in order to accommodate the conditon. To this point it has been secreting an excess of insulin to compensate for the Insulin Resistance. However, over time insulin production fails to such an extent that insulin injections are required, in which case the diabetic patient has progressed to Insulin Dependent Diabetes Mellitus. Note the cause is different from those who experience Insulin Dependent Diabetes Mellitus from childhood.

This phenomenon of Insulin Resistance is unfortunately becoming far too common in today's society. While the incidence of obesity (both childhood and adult) and diabetes continues to grow at frightening rates, so too does this interrelated but less well-known epidemic.

It is imperative to know that insulin resistance can act as a warning sign, heralding the onset of diabetes and other illnesses. If detected early, it can be appropriately managed and, in the majority of cases, full-blown diabetes can be prevented.

Ideally, fasting insulin levels should be less than or equal to 12 with a HOMA index less than 2.1. Such causes as consuming high glycemic load foods, high calorie and high bad fat diets, sedentary lifestyles, nutritional deficiencies, poorly managed stress, toxicity overload and hormones have all been implicated in the pathogenesis of Insulin Resistance and its consequences. It is easy to understand therefore why this is a disease of modern-day society.

Insulin Resistance has the potential to throw your body out of balance and affects the way your body regulates its fat and sugar levels. As previously stated, insulin itself is an anabolic hormone and a potent growth factor. This is why one of its early effects is fat storage and weight gain. This in turn is why it is intricately connected with other syndromes such as Metabolic Syndrome or Syndrome X, a cluster of co-occurring diseases that may include heart disease, diabetes, depression, and, in females, Polycystic Ovarian Syndrome

(PCOS).

Metabolic Syndrome involves an increase in abdominal girth (waist circumference >102cm in men and >88cm in women), an increase in fat around our abdominal organs, high blood pressure (>130/85), increased levels of triglycerides, low levels of HDL (good cholesterol) and elevated fasting glucose. It should be noted that abdominal girth measurements are debatable, and may vary for different populations. For example, the latest European values are >94cm for males and >80cm for females, while Asian values are >90cm for males and >80cm for females.

The ovaries are also sensitive to insulin. The higher levels of insulin that may be present change the rate of production of androgens (male hormones) in the ovaries. This in turn creates further hormonal imbalances, contributing to even higher levels of oestrogen, and hence oestrogen dominance. The latest evidence has also linked prostate cancer in men with the phenomenon of Insulin Resistance.

There are excellent books on Syndrome X (the Metabolic Syndrome) and PCOS already available on the shelf, so we are choosing to keep it simple and jump straight to management.

Lo and behold, dietary management is again one of the first principles to be upheld. As mentioned earlier, reducing your glycemic load, triglyceride and bad fat intake will make a significant difference.

Do the Food Elimination Regime as a kick-start to the Healthy Eating Plan. Once on the Healthy Eating Plan, additionally reduce (or even eradicate) your cereals/grains and non-starch vegetables for the following three months. Exercise is absolutely essential; 45 minutes per day! (Yes, you get an increase of 15 minutes if you have Insulin Resistance or Diabetes—get walking!). Weight loss and Insulin Resistance are intricately connected. **Weight loss will result in a decrease in insulin and a decrease in insulin will lead to weight loss.**

Exercise basically improves all aspects of the Metabolic Syndrome. It improves insulin sensitivity, decreases visceral (organ) fat and triglycerides, reduces VLDL, LDL and raises HDL cholesterol, reduces blood pressure and decreases thrombotic (clotting) tendencies. As mentioned earlier in the book, if you need help with exercise, enrol yourself in a gym program or get yourself a personal trainer.

If you know you are an emotional eater, then go back and re-read the section on managing your emotions. If you need more help, then seek out a counsellor or psychologist. For these issues need to be addressed if your quality of life is to be improved. And simply put, the earlier, the better. Remember that everyone needs help in at least one part of their lives at some time in their lives. It's all part of our respective life journeys.

So, what can you do from a nutritional perspective?

Chromium is a mineral absolutely essential for the production of Glucose Tolerance Factor (GTF). GTF is required to grease the lock that insulin opens, allowing glucose into the cell. It therefore has major effects on insulin sensitivity and carbohydrate metabolism. Many diabetics are deficient in this most important mineral. It is found in different foods including cereals such as wheat and rye (although you may need to eliminate or reduce these particular foods if Insulin Resistant), the root vegetables (carrots, potatoes, parsnips), apples, bananas, oranges, blueberries, peppers and spinach. Supplementation with a high dose of chromium picolinate (the most easily absorbed form of chromium) is also advised, combined with other nutrients, for a three month period.

Magnesium is another essential mineral in maintaining and improving both glucose and insulin homeostasis. By now, you should be aware of some of the most common symptoms of magnesium deficiency. Remember the eyelid twitches, heart palpitations, feelings of restlessness or restless legs, feelings of tightness or cramps in your legs and/ or feet and perhaps chocolate cravings (especially before periods)? If you do indeed experience these, then you should get a good response from magnesium supplementation.

Zinc also plays an essential role in the production, storage and secretion of insulin by the pancreatic islet cells.

Taurine is an amino acid that has been shown in many animal studies to reduce Insulin Resistance and hyper-triglyceridaemia, and also to prevent the accumulation of visceral fat. Similarly, lipoic acid also has a positive effect on Insulin Resistance.

There are several herbs, including cinnamon, fenugreek, gymnema and Panax ginseng, that have been shown in various studies to exert effects on glucose and/ or insulin homeostasis. Cinnamon is important for reducing levels of blood glucose, cholesterol and triglycerides while ginseng, fenugreek and gymnema perform similar roles for blood sugar regulation.

The following is a regime you may trial for three months if you have been diagnosed with Insulin Resistance, or impaired glucose tolerance or diabetes. Needless to say, this must be combined with an Insulin Resistance diet (Healthy Eating Plan with further reduction or complete exclusion of Cereal/ Grain and Starch Vegetable Groups) and consistent regular exercise.

INSULIN RESISTANCE & DIABETES MELLITUS

Chromium Picolinate	200-400ug in divided doses
Magnesium (elemental)	500mg
Zinc (elemental)	35-50mg
Taurine	1g in divided doses
Fenugreek	400mg
Gymnema Sylvestre	1g (leaf content)
Lipoic Acid	100mg

If your reason for Insulin Resistance is related to polycystic ovaries, then a herbal mix of vitex agnes castus, peony and liquorice may also be beneficial. We strongly suggest you seek professional assistance as PCOS is quite complicated and no one regime suits all.

Finally, it is essential to note that if you have been diagnosed by your doctor as having Diabetes Mellitus, you should be monitored by her or him on an ongoing basis, at least every three months. This is a medical condition requiring medical supervision, whether or not you need to use medication to manage it. If you are an early stage Non Insulin Dependent Diabetic, diet and exercise may be enough to control your disease, and if diligent enough, and with the support of nutritional supplementation, you may possibly reverse the underlying dysfunction.

If you are using medication and undertake a supplement program, again, your doctor needs to be informed. This is necessary even if your condition is improving, since if prescription medication dosages remain unchanged during your improvement, there is a risk of lowering blood sugar levels too far, leading to hypoglycemic complications.

If you are diabetic, be aware of what complications to look out for, both acute problems (blood sugar levels that are too high or too low) and in the long-term (eye problems, foot problems, kidney problems etc). Yet again a place for education from a doctor or Diabetic Educator.

Obesity and Resistant Weight Loss

You might be asking the question, am I obese? Let us just say, if you're asking the question, it's time to do something about your weight, regardless. Be honest, you're not likely to be asking the question if you're in well-toned condition.

To be slightly more scientific, here's a simple guide. Your Body Mass Index is equal to your weight in kilograms divided by your height in metres squared.

$$\text{Body Mass Index (BMI)} = \frac{\text{Mass (Kg)}}{\text{Height (m)} \times \text{Height (m)}}$$

Is it more than 25? Then you are drifting towards being overweight.

Is it more than 30? Time to definitely act.

Unless, of course, you are a musclebound lass or lad, and here is where BMI is not always accurate. It is a guide though (note that a BMI less than 20 indicates you're underweight).

So where do you begin if you have weight issues that have been resistant to dieting?

First of all, start with the Food Elimination Regime. In our experience most people will lose weight on this program. If you do not notice any loss in weight, it is time to consider the possible reasons why healthy eating is not leading to weight loss. And the most likely reasons revolve around whether or not you have one or more system dysfunctions that prevent you from losing weight.

THE THREE PREDOMINANT MEDICAL REASONS FOR NOT LOSING WEIGHT ARE CONSIDERED TO BE:

1. **Undiagnosed Insulin Resistance or Diabetes Mellitus (Type 2)**
2. **Hypothyroidism**
3. **Sex Hormone Imbalance (oestrogen dominance, progesterone deficiency)**

A good start would be to therefore read the chapters pertinent to these conditions in this book and see if they appear relevant to you.

There are also several other theorised and/or controversial medical reasons for a lack of weight loss that are less well researched. These include:

1. Poor digestive function
2. Liver toxicity (the need to 'detoxify' the liver first)
3. Pro-inflammatory body states
4. High stress levels (adrenal crisis and exhaustion)
5. Emotional Eating
6. Systemic Candida albicans infection.

Again, each of these subjects have a related chapter regarding potential supplementation in this section of the book. But it does pay to investigate whether they are pertinent to you, rather than take an all-out assault on supplementation based on assumption. The cost of the supplements will definitely add up and may not be necessary. Again, the more complicated your health needs, the greater the likelihood that a little money spent now on a professional consultation will save you a lot of money and time on potentially unnecessary supplements in the long-term. Money which could otherwise be spent on more essential needs (Health and Happiness).

The best advice therefore:

+ Before you buy a single supplement, get your diet and exercise programs stabilised first. If you are keen to accelerate weight loss, remove the cereal/grain and dairy groups from your diet for the first four to six weeks, taking a multivitamin to compensate for nutrient loss. Ultimately these food groups are not essential for your health **IF** you are eating appropriately from all other food groups (protein, fruits, vegetables and legumes/pulses) with particular emphasis on maximal vegetable intake.
+ Carefully consider undertaking the Food Elimination Regime during this period (with most cereals/grains and dairy being

therefore excluded anyway). Not only will it identify problem foods and aid gastrointestinal function, this regime also provides a period of 'detoxification' for the body as advocated by liver detoxification approaches to weight loss. Additionally, this is also an effective Insulin Resistance dietary approach, hence satisfactorily addressing several of the most likely medical reasons for an inability to lose weight.

✦ The only exception to this would be if Systemic Candida Albicans Infection is suspected. In this case, more strict dietary approaches are advocated with an initial elimination of all fruits and additional vegetables from the diet. This is perhaps the most controversial argument for lack of weight loss, but in the presence of indicative signs and symptoms (see Chapter 10 of this section, 'Creating a Healthy Immune System'), it might be considered.

✦ If you cannot commit to any eating plan, investigate the reasons for your lack of commitment. If you are emotionally eating, first investigate what is driving your self-sabotage or lack of motivation before any further commitments are made.

✦ If considering supplements, address all health concerns first before focusing specifically on supplementing for weight loss.

✦ Unless other medical conditions are obviously of priority, start with nutrients directed towards Insulin Resistance first. These include magnesium, B Complex, zinc, chromium as well as lipoic acid, in the dosages recommended in this chapter.

✦ Investigate other reasons for slow weight loss through the Dysfunctions and Disease questions at the start of the following chapters.
   (i)   Gastrointestinal Health (Chapter 2)
   (ii) Demystifying the Liver (Chapter 3)
   (iii) Hormone Health (Chapter 7)
   (iv) Neurotransmitter Health (Chapter 8)
   (v)   Creating a Healthy Immune System (Chapter 10)

✦ Do not depend excessively on supplementation. Investigate one or two systems at a time and begin first with the dietary recommendations rather than supplementation approaches. Choose what appears most important with the aid of the questions at the start of the chapter, or with the help of a doctor or other health professional.

Remember, diet and exercise first ... only after which should you consider supplementation!

7

Hormone Health

There are many who may have flicked straight to this section because you know how great an influence hormones hold over you, controlling your life in so many different ways. If this is you, we advise you to take only a cursory glance at this chapter, then return to the start of the book. Why? Because our hormones themselves are also affected just as much by our other life circumstances, such as our thoughts, our stress levels, our diets and so on, as they in turn affect the remainder of our lives.

On the other hand, you may be an individual whose hormones are currently in perfect balance. Wonderful! However, it is important for you to know just how much hormones can control the life of a person who may in fact be your partner, your sibling, your parent or your child. No doubt someone in your family will have their lives afflicted with hormonal imbalances. Like everything else in life, it helps to understand, it helps to empathise, it helps to offer assistance when things seem totally out of control.

And when it comes to hormones, this is exactly what all too often happens!

So, on that note, let's see which hormones are those primarily responsible for exerting such strong influences over our lives. We can basically break them into several groups. Please note that these groups are in no way complete or mutually exclusive but we are aiming, of course, to keep it simple!

1. **Our Reproductive Hormones**
   Including Oestrogen, Progesterone, Testosterone
2. **Our Thyroid Hormones**
   Including TSH (thyroid stimulating hormone), Free T4, Free T3
3. **Our Steroid Hormones**
   Including DHEA (Dihydroepiandrostenedione), Cortisone, Adrenaline, Noradrenaline
4. **Our Brain Hormones (Neurotransmitters)**
   Including Serotonin, Dopamine, GABA (Gamma Amino Butyric Acid), Melatonin, Histamine
5. **Our Anabolic and Catabolic Hormones**
   Including Insulin (see previous chapter) and Growth Hormone

From the start, it is vital to reiterate that these are simply the most commonly known and studied hormones. New hormones and new binding globulins (substances that can inactivate these hormones) are being discovered every day. As this is not designed to be a formal medical textbook devoted to hormones, but rather an action handbook, we will simply discuss those relevant points that may further your understanding of your own hormones and possibly guide you towards creating better balance. Many hormones cannot yet be directly measured through pathology tests and therefore potential diagnoses depend purely on clinical acumen and experience.

Obviously, this does require professional assistance; however, there are many hormones that depend simply on nutrients for their ongoing production and optimal function.

And believe it or not, the simple addition of previously deficient nutrients can make an absolutely amazing difference to our general health and wellbeing.

So, let's begin the journey!

Our Reproductive Hormones

YOU SHOULD CONSIDER THE FOLLOWING ADVICE REGARDING FEMALE HORMONES IF:

You are menstruating and have:

Irregular or No Periods	**Yes / No**
Light or Heavy Periods	**Yes / No**

You experience PMT including:

Mood Changes	**Yes / No**
Breast Tenderness	**Yes / No**
Headaches	**Yes / No**
Sinus Problems	**Yes / No**
Chocolate Cravings	**Yes / No**

If you are not having periods:

Hot Flushes	**Yes / No**
Night Sweats	**Yes / No**
Palpitations	**Yes / No**
Insomnia	**Yes / No**
Mood Changes	**Yes / No**
Loss of Libido	**Yes / No**
Lack of Energy	**Yes / No**

Diagnosable Syndromes or Diseases specifically involving Reproductive Hormones include:

- Pre-Menstrual Syndrome, Perimenopausal or Menopausal Symptoms
- Endometriosis, Polycystic Ovary Disease, Infertility, Ovarian and Breast Cysts

In our practice, an imbalance of oestrogens and progesterone is by far the most common culprit when it comes to hormone problems. This means, in particular, an excess of oestrogen (oestrogen dominance) compared with a progesterone deficiency. Most nutritionists, naturopaths and nutritionally oriented medical doctors would definitely agree.

This can arise from a multitude of causes (many being controversial, of course) including xeno-oestrogens (substances that mimic oestrogen, found in plastic water bottles exposed to the sun, for example), an excess of copper in the body (via contaminated soils and water pipes) and the use of hormones in the commercial farming of animals. As generations continue, this is unfortunately likely to progress further as many of these substances can stay in the body and even change our genetic code.

So let's discuss the possible symptoms and consequences.

Oestrogen Dominance or Progesterone Deficiency: One and the Same

From the start, it is important to clarify that it is the ratio between oestrogen and progesterone that is most significant. As no man is an island, no hormone stands alone either. Increasing one of the sex hormones will decrease the other and vice versa, and it is the relative balance that matters. This is an important concept to be remembered.

Oestrogen dominance or progesterone deficiency occurs primarily in women who are menstruating, from pubertal girls through to perimenopausal women. These are women who experience problems with their periods and premenstrual symptoms of any nature.

In the menstruating woman the following signs and symptoms are pertinent:
- Heavy periods
- Prolonged periods

- Clots with periods
- Painful periods
- Dark blood spotting prior to menstrual flow
- Breakthrough spotting or bleeding at ovulation
- Premenstrual breast tenderness
- Premenstrual headaches
- Premenstrual mood changes
- Premenstrual sinus problems
- Premenstrual joint aches
- Premenstrual chocolate cravings

Primarily in the perimenopausal or menopausal woman:
- Vagueness, irrationality
- Over-reacting for little or often no reason
- Heart palpitations
- Insomnia
- Hot flushes (sometimes these are related to oestrogen deficiency)
- Loss of bone mineral density (also secondary to oestrogen deficiency)
- Generalised aches and pains

It is important to note that the above symptoms can and do occur in women who have had a hysterectomy, if their ovaries are still intact. In fact, often the underlying reason for the hysterectomy was actually oestrogen dominance. Conditions such as fibroids, endometriosis, dysfunctional prolonged bleeding, polycystic ovarian disease (PCO), fibrous breast tissue, breast cysts and oestrogen dependent breast cancers are almost always connected with an excess of oestrogen.

Like most other clinical pictures, oestrogen dominance occurs as a continuum, ranging from simple PMT to complicated conditions such as PCO. For this reason, it is advisable to consult a professional who can exclude the main concerns, so to speak (PCO, cancer). Mostly, this is done by ultrasound (pelvic, breast) with a mammogram as necessary. It should be noted that endometriosis cannot be detected by ultrasound and actually currently requires a laparoscopy for diagnosis.

In many cases, oestrogen dominance can be lessened with symptoms subsequently improved. Generally speaking, though, the worse the imbalance, the harder the task.

So, what can YOU do?

Many women with progesterone deficiency are also deficient in magnesium as this vitamin is necessary to produce progesterone. There are five simple questions to determine if you have magnesium deficiency.

Do you experience:
- Eyelid or other body twitches?
- Heart palpitations (in the absence of cardiac disease)?
- Restlessness or restless legs?
- Feelings of tightness or cramps in your legs or feet?
- Chocolate cravings, particularly before periods?

If you have answered 'yes' to any one of these questions, then you are very likely to be suffering with a degree of magnesium deficiency. If this is the case, then these symptoms should disappear once on a supplement.

It is important to highlight that nutritional medicine does not work overnight and this may take several months, even with supplementation. So eyelid twitches don't bother you. That's understandable, but it is simply your body's way of telling you that you need a particular nutrient. Here is a good time to also remember how complex the body is. Magnesium is certainly not only needed to produce progesterone. Rather, magnesium is actually required for over 500 different reactions in our bodies, each being necessary to maintain optimal health and wellbeing.

Furthermore, it takes a healthy digestive system to be able to absorb and actually use such nutrients. So can you see why we discussed digestion at the very beginning of this section? Its importance is astounding!

As well as magnesium, vitamins such as B6 are also needed to increase progesterone levels. Pyridoxal-5-phosphate is the physiologically active form of B6 and the body must be able to convert regular B6 into this form if this is not directly supplemented. It is also important to know that one can become toxic with excess levels of vitamin B6, the first sign often being pins and needles in the hands or feet. This is reversible if the dose is reduced or ceased accordingly. As you already know, it is also necessary to take a B complex whenever taking a specific B vitamin in order to avoid competition between the B vitamins.

Vitex agnes castus (commonly known as chastetree or chasteberry) is a herb that has been used for many centuries in order to help those afflicted with hormonal imbalances. And with good effects. Accordingly, it is now among the ever-increasing body of herbs that are being studied in the name of evidence-based medicine. Vitex has been shown to act on dopamine, oestrogen, progesterone and, most recently, opiate receptors.

A 2005 systematic review concluded that Vitex is a safe herbal medicine and no drug interactions have been reported. However, it may theoretically counteract the effect of dopamine agonist and antagonist drugs. It is important to ask your GP if you are not sure if you are taking such a drug. As it is a hormone modulator, Vitex is not recommended for people with hormone dependent tumours, or in pregnancy, until safety for these conditions has been established.

In our clinical experience, Vitex works a treat when combined with magnesium and Vitamin B6 in reducing oestrogen dominance. Remember, the regime will have some effect in the first month, more effect in the second and maximum effect in the third. After this time, you can play with your regime. Like in many other cases, now that you are aware, your body will simply tell you when it's deficient and needing more. Take note that just as it takes three months to achieve optimal levels on any one regime, it will take up to three months for you to truly feel your new base level without supplementation.

OESTROGEN DOMINANCE/PROGESTERONE INSUFFICIENCY

Magnesium (elemental)	500mg
B Complex	
Vitamin B6	100mg
Vitex Agnus Castus	1000–2000mg before breakfast

The above doses are given only as a guide. Your results will depend upon your own level of compliance, where in the spectrum of imbalance you fall and the quality of your supplements. Like most things in life, you generally get what you pay for.

As an added point, foods are of course a wonderful source of nutrients. However, when there are deficiencies present, nutritional supplementation is almost always required in order to achieve earlier results. Once reached, maintenance levels can generally provided through different food groups.

The authors understand that there certainly are other means of balancing such hormones through the use of homeopathy and the like, but we are simply choosing to share that which works best in our own experience.

If, after three months, you feel that results could be better, we advise you to seek professional advice if you have not already, to perform any relevant investigations and consider the use of any stronger substances, such as bio-identical or natural hormones. The latter are a viable alternative option where nutritional supplementation has not been effective, but they can only be accessed via a doctor's prescription (you will need to find a nutritionally orientated doctor in most instances for this) and through a compounding chemist, so further words are wasted here.

Oestrogen Deficiency

The vast majority of women who suffer from oestrogen deficiency are older perimenopausal or post-menopausal women. The main complaints are vaginal dryness, hot flushes, skin dryness and a loss of bone mineral density, known as osteopaenia when mild and osteoporosis when moderate or worse. **As an aside, there are no symptoms of osteoporosis hence every perimenopausal woman should be screened for bone loss**. In our practice, approximately one out of four women at this time in their lives are shown to have osteopaenia. In other words, are on their way towards osteoporosis.

In regard to the latter, bone mineral density tests are only recommended two-yearly, but there are tests available (Urinary N-Telopeptides) that allow you to have some idea of whether the treatment you are on is having an effect or not after six months (see 'Bones, Joints and Muscles', Chapter 9 of this section). Generally, a good bone supplement will do the trick.

Sometimes, bio-identical hormones or other drugs may be necessary. Needless to say, a good diet, being smoke-free and regular weight-bearing exercises will work hand in hand to optimise your bone strength (noting that a slow decline in bone strength is a normal feature of ageing).

For many women, vaginal dryness can be overcome by the use of simple lubricants. Alternatively, compounding chemists can make Vitamin E pessaries in coconut oil, for example, which also serve to overcome the problem in many cases. Oestrogen type creams can be used, but the use of unopposed oestrogens is certainly controversial and not recommended long term.

Hot flushes may be a symptom of either progesterone or oestrogen deficiency. There are often triggers such as alcohol that should be identified in order to minimise the frequency of flushes. The use of certain herbs such as black cohosh may certainly help the majority of women. In our own clinical experiences, no adversely affected liver function tests have been seen after administration of black cohosh; however, it should be noted that there will soon be warnings on any herbal medications containing black cohosh stating that it may adversely affect the liver in some people, so be aware of this risk, however small.

There are many over-the-counter preparations designed to reduce the symptoms of perimenopause and menopause, but different preparations work for different women. Our advice is to take the maximum recommended dosage for two-three months and then judge your own response. If they have a limited or unsatisfactory effect, try another. If this fails, seek professional advice.

For problems with dry skin related to oestrogen deficiency, we find that essential fatty acids (EFA) for three-six months will generally help. The underlying cause is usually EFA deficiency. Look for brittle nails and rough goose-flesh skin on the upper arms and you have clinched the diagnosis in one. Remember that these cosmetic concerns are indicative of a general inadequacy of omega-3 oils throughout the body, which should not be ignored.

A nutritionally orientated doctor has the option of bio-identical hormones when other nutritional options either fail to have effect, or where more intense approaches are indicated. Let it be said that the use of hormones, be they bio-identical or natural, should be limited to the lowest doses and used only when absolutely necessary. Often they may be trialled for a short period of time to assess effect, and where possible, weaned once positive results have been achieved.

Testosterone

Males AND Females can experience testosterone imbalance so you should take note if:

You lack sex drive	Yes / No
You suffer from impotency (men)	Yes / No
You lack sexual stamina	Yes / No
Your hair is prematurely thinning	Yes / No
You have previously used anabolic steroids	Yes / No
You are a woman with excess facial and/or body hair with irregular periods	Yes / No

There are several important points that need to be made regarding testosterone. Like all other hormones, both men and women produce testosterone. Testosterone levels may be high or low. They are best determined through blood tests which measure the levels of free androgens (FAI- Free Androgen Index) or by salivary hormone tests.

Testosterone is generally associated with libido or sex drive, and low libido is extremely common.

BUT LOW LIBIDO DOES NOT NECESSARILY MEAN LOW TESTOSTERONE!

A lack of libido in women is definitely multi-factorial in the majority of cases, meaning that simple testosterone replacement and supplementation alone may not improve the situation. Men who lack energy, sex drive and/or muscle tone and notice their behaviour is changing may certainly be deficient in testosterone and other hormones such as DHEA (see Adrenal Hormones). This generally occurs around mid-life (andropause) but can occur at any time. If you think you are in this category, have your levels of testosterone, DHEA checked. It can certainly make a huge difference to your life if appropriately treated!

Given this, supplements that may help with low testosterone include Omega-3 essential fatty acids (EPA/DHA), zinc, selenium and Vitamin C due to their importance in testosterone synthesis. But to repeat, before taking such supplementation ensure that you are actually low in testosterone to begin with.

TESTOSTERONE SUPPORT

Omega-3 fish oils EPA/ DHA	4g
Vitamin C	3g
Selenium (elemental)	150ug
Zinc (elemental)	35–50mg (bedtime)

Note that many women with low libido actually have high testosterone levels! We therefore also recommend you have your testosterone levels checked before embarking on the use of any type of testosterone enhancing program. It can be dangerous to play with your hormones.

If you are concerned about your libido (male or female) there are many over-the-counter preparations designed to improve it (including Arginine, Tribulus and the excitingly named Horny Goat Weed ... as long as you are a goat!). This is obviously an area ripe for many and varied claims. If you want to explore supplements, try taking the maximum dose of a product as directed for two months and then judge for yourself.

More often than not, the cause for low libido is multi-factorial and there often needs to be some form of active communication, participation and pact involving both partners over this time to determine the true cause (is it physical, psychological, related to relationship problems or a combination of all?). Please note that impotency may in fact be an indication for other serious illnesses, such as Diabetes Mellitus. Therefore we strongly recommend you consult your doctor if you suffer with this problem.

IMPROVING LIBIDO

Arginine*   3g
Tribulus and/or Horny goat weed as directed

Also helps with Impotency and Premature Ejaculation but increases likelihood of cold sores/herpes if susceptible. Also not recommended without a doctor's advice if you suffer with any cardiovascular disease.

Women who have Polycystic Ovarian Syndrome (PCOS) may have an imbalance of testosterone. In PCO, testosterone levels are usually high. As mentioned earlier, other hormones are also out of balance. Symptoms of PCO may include irregular periods, acne, excess facial or body hair, problems conceiving, unstable moods and weight gain. The diagnosis can generally be made through blood tests (FAI, SHBG –Sex Hormone Binding Globulin, fasting insulin) and a pelvic ultrasound. Professional advice from a nutritionally orientated doctor or naturopath is certainly recommended.

Suffice it to say that with the correct program individually designed for you, good results may be achieved within three months. You may find some improvement with the regime to increase your body's progesterone, but often after an individually tailored herbal mix is added.

The Thyroid Hormones

Our thyroid gland exerts a major influence on so many body systems. It can be working perfectly or possibly functioning in either an underactive or overactive fashion.

Hypothyroidism

Consider the possibility of Hypothyroidism* if:

You have noticed a steady increase in your weight without a change in diet	Yes / No
You have noticed hair falling out	Yes / No
You are finding cold weather increasingly discomforting	Yes / No

Your eyebrows are thinning	**Yes / No**
You find it hard to get going in the morning	**Yes / No**
You are depressed	**Yes / No**
You are generally lethargic	**Yes / No**
You have low libido	**Yes / No**
You are constipated	**Yes / No**

*Please note the overlap of such symptoms with an imbalance in many other systems.

Hypothyroidism or underactive thyroid is by far the most common pathology.

There are several possible causes including genetics, stress, auto-immune disorders and viral infections.

Symptoms may include fatigue, weight gain, hair loss, flat or depressed moods, cold peripheries, poor libido, constipation, and the list goes on. It is important to understand that many of these symptoms may also occur with different hormone imbalances or other more complex conditions. It is generally more common in women but can certainly happen in men.

One of the best ways to exclude low thyroid function is by measuring your core temperature. The thermometer is best left beside your bed whilst you are sleeping then, first thing in the morning, before you get out of bed, take your temperature with the thermometer under your tongue. Do this for three mornings. If you are still menstruating or ovulating, you need to do this either during your periods or shortly after. For as you ovulate, your temperature rises and this will give you a false reading. Temperatures below 36.0c are very suspicious of an underactive thyroid, with temperatures at 36.3c being fairly normal.

If your temperatures are low or you have symptoms with a family history of thyroid diseases, it is worthwhile having your blood checked. The most beneficial test is a Free T3 level (FT3), as this is the physiologically active form of thyroid hormone. TSH (thyroid stimulating hormone) and Free T4 will almost always be tested but some pathology labs will not perform a FT3 level if the TSH level is considered normal (<5.0). Many nutritionally orientated doctors consider a TSH level above 2.0 to be suspicious of an underactive thyroid. If this is the case, private pathology laboratories can perform Free T3 levels for a reasonable price. Thyroid antibodies may also be tested to confirm the presence of Hashimoto's or Graves' disease.

There is another important concept that you should understand. When you are stressed, the body makes more of another hormone called Reverse T3, which is basically inactive, instead of producing FT3. Here the significance of the Mindbody continuum is again highlighted. RT3 can be measured by private laboratories; however, the results take many weeks and usually the patient can tell if they are stressed or not for free! The bottom line is, the more Reverse T3 rather than FT3, the less effective your thyroid output.

The following is a regime that we use in our practice to support a low-functioning thyroid.

LOW THYROID FUNCTION

Tyrosine in divided doses	1000mg
Selenium (elemental)	150ug bedtime
Kelp (containing Iodine)	1–2g
Zinc (elemental)	35–50mg bedtime if deficient

Tyrosine, iodine, selenium and zinc are some of the co-factors necessary for the conversion of inactive FT4 to active FT3. This regime should be trialled for three months and one's temperature recorded again at the end of this trial. Patients can judge for themselves any particular benefits, such as more energy and wellbeing, better digestion and improved moods. Seaweed and other iodine rich foods can also be helpful.

If further improvement is desired, then professional consultation is necessary for the possibility of replacing thyroid hormone in the form of either thyroxine or a slow-release preparation of FT3, which is only available by prescription from compounding chemists.

Hyperthyroidism

Consider discussing hyperthyroidism (or the symptoms of hyperthyroidism) with your doctor if:

You have noticed unexplainable and rapid weight loss	Yes / No
You have noticed heart palpitations or anxiety	Yes / No
You have noted an unexplainable increase in appetite	Yes / No
You have become markedly sensitive to warm weather	Yes / No
You have noticed a significant change in your moods	Yes / No

Hyperthyroidism is a serious condition that must involve the assistance of a medical doctor and/ or endocrinologist to treat. Blood tests, thyroid ultrasounds and thyroid nuclear scans may all be necessary and the treatment almost always involves pharmaceutical medications, rather than only nutritional support. Graves' Disease is the most common reason for an overactive thyroid and involves very high levels of thyroid antibodies. An overactive thyroid makes a person feel anxious and speedy, experience heart palpitations and diarrhoea. They are very hungry yet continue to lose weight and they are basically very unwell. If this is you, then see your doctor immediately to exclude an overactive thyroid.

Adrenal Support and DHEA (Dihydroepiandrostenedione)
You may be in need of adrenal support if:

You have been chronically stressed	Yes / No
You suffer from mood swings	Yes / No
You experience decreased energy and wellbeing	Yes / No
You feel stressed without reason	Yes / No
You are overly anxious or startle easily	Yes / No

… **and additionally have answered positively to questions regarding other hormonal imbalances, which may instead reflect Adrenal Exhaustion.**

If you are under stress, and as a consequence experiencing adrenal exhaustion, you may need to support your DHEA production (Dihydroepiandrostenodine). DHEA is produced in the adrenal gland from another hormone called pregnenolone, which is itself derived from cholesterol. DHEA is one of our main energy producing hormones, with both adrenaline and noradrenaline being created as its sons and daughters later on in the hormone cascade.

DHEA is known to decrease with age and with illness. It is therefore sometimes referred to as an 'anti-ageing hormone'. The most prevalent symptom of low DHEA is fatigue and lack of wellbeing. Lack of libido is also a significant symptom.

It can be measured by blood or saliva, with saliva being the generally preferred method. In our clinical experience, the results are fairly similar.

If energy is down and/or DHEA is low, certain nutrients and herbs can be used to help boost one's energy. Such herbs include ginseng and gingko, providing there are no contraindications such as with anti-clotting medications (eg. Warfarin). As always, check with your GP or pharmacist regarding such interactions. Other supportive nutrients include tyrosine, all the B Vitamin group, and Vitamin C. A broad spectrum multivitamin and Co-Enzyme Q10 may also be helpful if you want to completely cover the needs of your adrenal gland.

ADRENAL SUPPORT

Ginseng	1–2g
Gingko biloba	500–1000mg
Tyrosine	1000mg
B Complex	
Magnesium (elemental)	500mg divided
Vitamin C	3g
Plus ...	
Broad spectrum multivitamin and if required Co-Enzyme Q10	100–200mg

As an aside, remember common things occur commonly. Fatigue may also be due to other deficiencies. Before resorting to solely trying to increase your DHEA levels, make sure you have your ferritin or iron stores (see Chapter 4) and Vitamin B12 levels checked by blood test. Nutritional doctors disagree with the range of normal blood levels of these nutrients suggested by some pathology laboratories. The range of Vitamin B12 is generally considered to be between 130–1500, with an ideal level being midway around 800.

Unlike iron, one cannot become toxic with Vitamin B12. Remember, though, that a B Complex (including folate) is essential to take with any one B vitamin to avoid competition between the other B vitamins. Alternatively, if your doctor is amenable, consider a course of Vitamin B12 injections (1–10mg/dose for 6 doses).

LOW B12 LEVELS (3 MONTHS)

Vitamin B12   1000ug
Plus additional B Complex

Furthermore, check your temperatures: an underactive thyroid will also need to be excluded. Excessive stress and/or workload, poor sleep and poor digestion are other common reasons for fatigue besides low DHEA.

If all these are normal and any other underlying pathology associated with more serious diseases excluded, and supplementation has not provided you with any benefit, then it is possible to work at supporting your adrenal function with DHEA as a bio-identical hormone under close supervision of a qualified medical practitioner. Again, you may need to seek out a nutritionally orientated medical practitioner who is willing to give this a try. But it may well be worth it if you are to be able to return from a stressful and fatigued state of being to the vibrant healthy Self you wish to be.

Human Growth Hormone

Here is a very short note on human growth hormone (HGH), added because many may have heard of it due to its association with anti-ageing. There are indeed some individuals with excessively low levels of growth hormone and these people may indeed benefit from Human Growth Hormone injections. The primary tests to confirm deficiency of Human Growth Hormone are blood tests called IGF-1 and IGF-BP3. If these are low, then we strongly advise you to see a medical practitioner trained in administering growth hormone therapies.

For the majority of people, however, Human Growth Hormone can be increased naturally. Participation in a resistance exercise program as typified by gym based training will automatically encourage the production of HGH.

Caloric restriction and a high quality protein powder containing serious quantities of the amino acids arginine, ornithine, tyrosine, glutathione and methionine will also improve natural HGH production. This combination is certainly going to make you feel younger anyway, so why not give healthy hyper-living a try? Combine this with a serious application to meditation and self-development and you're more than halfway there!

8

Neurotransmitter Health

The following chapter may be particularly relevant to you if:

You are experiencing depression	Yes / No
You are anxious or experience stress easily	Yes / No
You find it hard to relax	Yes / No
You have a diagnosed mental health condition	Yes / No
You have poor concentration	Yes / No
You find it difficult to motivate yourself	Yes / No
You feel out of rhythm with the time of day	Yes / No
You have an overactive mind	Yes / No
You use recreational drugs, alcohol, caffeine or nicotine to cope with emotions you otherwise find difficult to deal with	Yes / No
You find it difficult to control your actions	Yes / No

Diagnosable diseases specifically involving neurotransmitter balance include:

- ✦ Depression, Anxiety, Panic Attacks
- ✦ Schizophrenia, Obsessive Compulsive and Bipolar Affective Disorder
- ✦ Autism, Attention Deficit Disorder, Learning Disabilities
- ✦ Migraine and other Headaches

Our neurotransmitters are basically our brain's messengers. They have up until the last few decades been thought to have only been produced in the brain.

On the contrary, it is now known that many of our neurotransmitters also play roles as hormones in the digestive system and are called 'Neuro-Gut Peptides'. Not only can they be made outside the central nervous system, these peptides can and do travel throughout the body, continually exerting their influence on other hormones and other systems, such as the immune system.

Hence the new medical fields of Psychoneuroimmunology and Psychoneuroendocrinology, for example. As we are keeping it simple, suffice it to say that these transmitters, these hormones, these peptides, are extremely powerful in their control of the human body. To remind you once again, we are at the very least a MindBody Continuum.

Healthy body, healthy mind ... Healthy mind, healthy body.

As mentioned previously, more and more of these neurotransmitters, neurochemicals and hormones are being discovered every day, and their effects are continuing to be researched throughout the world.

We have chosen to focus on a few major well-known neurotransmitters in keeping with the simple concept of this book. Always remember, though, that you are a complex Being and every thought, every intent, every action has the potential to create a 'butterfly effect' throughout your entire Universe!

Serotonin

Most of you would have heard of serotonin. It is colloquially termed one of our 'happy hormones'. Pharmaceutical medications that stop the breakdown of serotonin in our brains and bodies are called anti-depressant drugs. This alone serves to highlight why adequate levels of serotonin in the brain are essential for optimal health and happiness.

Simply put, it is a serotonin deficiency that may be present in our brains when depressed rather than an anti-depressant deficiency!

When we are happy, serotonin creation is naturally reinforced. Yet when things go wrong in life, or wrong in our production of serotonin, we may need to give our brains a helping hand. How can we do this?

Serotonin itself is derived from an amino acid called tryptophan. No doubt you have heard the old wives' tale of having a glass of warm milk before bed in order to help you sleep. This is because milk contains tryptophan and another known function of serotonin is in fact to help with sleep disturbances via its conversion to melatonin. It is important to note that tryptophan itself requires several co-factors to assist it in its conversion to serotonin. These include Vitamin B6, zinc, iron, calcium, Vitamin C, folic acid and vitamin B3.

It is interesting to note that Vitamin B6 and zinc have been found to be needed in almost all chemical reactions involving brain neurotransmitters and basic mental health.

Scary when you are aware of the actual incidence of zinc deficiency in the world population! The Pfeiffer Institute in the United States has one of the most extensive databases in the world comprising of blood, urine and saliva samples that have been studied to further increase our knowledge in this field. It is important to know that these studies have revealed that almost all individuals with some form of mental health issue, ranging from depression, schizophrenia and bipolar disease through to the autistic spectrum disorders, have a deficiency in zinc and/or vitamin B6.

So to a lesson in simple biochemistry, if only to reinforce why the sceptics of nutritional medicines should think again about their anti-supplementation arguments. Consume protein and you consume tryptophan. But that doesn't automatically mean we will make serotonin. We still need to convert this to 5 Hydroxy-tryptophan then in turn to serotonin. And both steps require nutrients to take place effectively.

If we do not have the nutrients it simply won't happen. So to make it happen, supply more nutrients. Supplement with folic acid, calcium, Vitamin C, iron, and, in turn, Vitamin B6 and zinc. What about the other pathway leading to Vitamin B3? This is important, too, but only if you have insufficient Vitamin B3. Why? Because otherwise, tryptophan may take this path instead, leaving less to make serotonin.

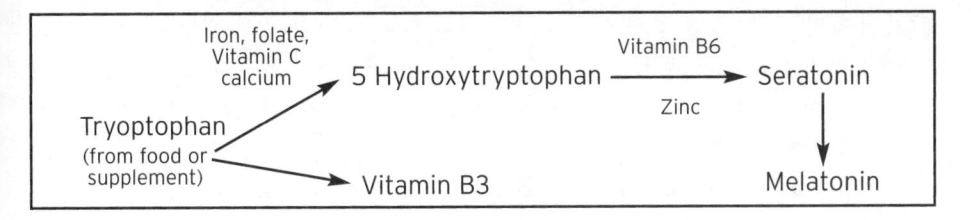

```
                    Iron, folate,              Vitamin B6
                    Vitamin C
                      calcium  → 5 Hydroxytryptophan ─────→ Seratonin
    Tryoptophan                              Zinc               │
    (from food or                                               ↓
     supplement)          → Vitamin B3                      Melatonin
```

There you go, your own simple lesson in the science of balancing some of your brain's neurotransmitters. It is a little more complicated than this, but let's face it, you now understand the nutritional supplementation approach to neurotransmitters far better than most. So let us see how this applies to other neurotransmitters.

Dopamine, Adrenaline, Noradrenaline

Dopamine has become fairly well known due to its connection with Parkinson's Disease (deficiency of dopamine) and schizophrenia (excess of dopamine). Of course, both conditions have a multitude of other causes and imbalances, but this is not the point here. Dopamine is also referred to as a positive inotrope and is used extensively in Intensive Care Units in order to support the cardiovascular system. It has been found to have a major role in working memory and its deficiency has recently been implicated in both depression and alcohol and drug addiction. Just to highlight the plethora of different roles each of these neurotransmitters play in our incredibly complex human bodies.

Dopamine is derived from tyrosine, an amazing amino acid that, as you might remember, is also necessary for the production of FT3 (thyroid hormone, as mentioned previously). Tyrosine is also required for the production of adrenaline and noradrenaline through the hormone DHEA. Needless to say, all three neurotransmitters are vital to our health and wellbeing. So, how do you supplement to increase your dopamine levels and in turn adrenaline and noradrenaline?

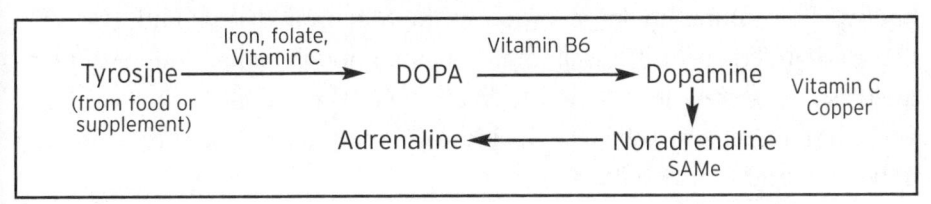

```
                 Iron, folate,         Vitamin B6
                  Vitamin C
    Tyrosine ─────────────→ DOPA ─────────────→ Dopamine    Vitamin C
    (from food or                                   │         Copper
     supplement)                                    ↓
                       Adrenaline ←──────── Noradrenaline
                                              SAMe
```

GABA

GABA is the main inhibitory neurotransmitter in the brain. This means it has the ability to turn other neurotransmitters off or at least modulate their effect where necessary.

Therefore a deficiency of GABA has been implicated in anxiety, panic attacks, epilepsy and insomnia: all conditions where there is an inability to switch off the mind and/or the body. Pharmaceutical drugs used for the above conditions are designed to assist the function of GABA receptors in the brain.

You will not be surprised to learn that GABA is derived from yet another amino acid, glutamine. As amino acids are, indeed, the building blocks of protein, you can see why we devoted time earlier in the book to the importance of having a healthy digestive system and a healthy diet containing, importantly, a moderate level of protein.

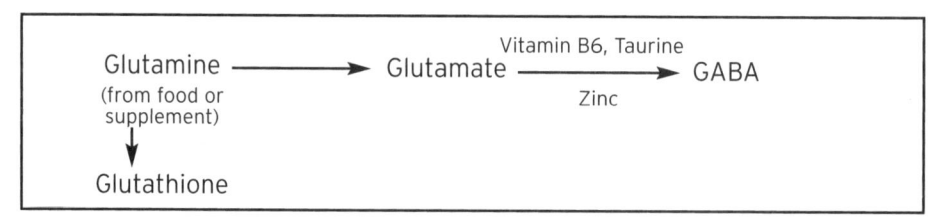

```
                                    Vitamin B6, Taurine
    Glutamine  ──────▶  Glutamate  ──────────────▶  GABA
    (from food or                        Zinc
    supplement)
        │
        ▼
    Glutathione
```

It should be noted that glutamate is an excitatory neurotransmitter and therefore a deficiency of the co-factors zinc, Vitamin B6 and taurine will cause more glutamate to build up and subsequently trigger the above symptoms. It is therefore vitally important that we are able to turn glutamate into GABA if want to be able to relax!

Note again that supplementation needs to be functional rather than single shot nutrient doses if it is to work effectively.

As mentioned, the other derivative from glutamine, glutathione, is a very powerful antioxidant essential to the functioning of every cell in our bodies. It is found in large amounts in the brain tissue and becomes depleted in times of stress if there is not enough glutamine present to replenish its stores. It is therefore vitally important to note that we need enough glutamine to satisfy both sides of the equation if we are to remain in healthy and happy balance.

Histamine

We are all aware of antihistamine drugs that help in the treatment of allergic reactions, hay fever and the like. But histamine itself is involved in a multitude of other actions in the body. For instance, it supports the cardiovascular system by regulating blood pressure and promotes the secretion of hydrochloric acid in the stomach. Low levels of histidine (the amino acid precursor to histamine) have also been found in the blood and synovial (joint) fluid in patients with rheumatoid arthritis.

Furthermore, histamine increases the release of serotonin and imbalances of histamine may contribute to increased anxiety levels and schizophrenia. In fact, there are now different classifications for schizophrenia emerging, according to whether an individual is actually histopaenic (deficient in histamine) or histadelic (excess of histamine).

How do we turn the amino acid histidine into histamine? Again, the importance of Vitamin B6 cannot be over estimated.

$$\text{Histadine (from food or supplement)} \xrightarrow{\text{Vitamin B6}} \text{Histamine}$$

Melatonin

Melatonin is the dark twin of serotonin, for as day turns to night, some of your brain's serotonin is converted into melatonin by the pineal gland. Receptors in the eyes alert the pineal gland to changes in light, switching it on when dark to the process of creating melatonin.

Melatonin is important as it acts to some degree as a master hormone, regulating other hormones through its action on our body's natural biorhythms. Not only do we begin to tire and get ready for sleep because of melatonin, but every organ, tissue and cell in our body responds to night-day patterns with its own change in performance as appropriate. In effect the pineal gland, through its production of melatonin, is our body's own biological clock that keeps us in rhythm with our requirements for activity and sleep during different parts of the day and night.

Melatonin has been linked to healthy ageing. It is a powerful antioxidant, maintains a healthy immune system, has cancer fighting properties and, of course, plays a major role in sleep regulation (including combating jet lag). Deficiencies of melatonin may cause inappropriate tiredness during the day, wakefulness at night, sleep disturbances, difficulty concentrating, memory disturbances and unexplained changes in sleep activity.

Melatonin can either be prescribed by a nutritionally orientated doctor or taken via homeopathics. Nutritional supplementation as for serotonin will also help for melatonin due to the close relationship. But first of all you might need to decide whether supplementing is putting the cart before the horse. It may actually be your lifestyle choices causing melatonin deficiency, rather than melatonin deficiency to begin with. How so? Well, let's look at what might cause melatonin imbalances:

- Ageing (this isn't your fault)
- Office work (fluorescent lighting)
- Excess exercise
- Shift work
- Smoking
- Exposure to electromagnetic fields (electric blankets including that in a waterbed, fluorescent lighting, computer monitors, copiers and printers etc)
- Increased free radical exposure through air pollutants, chemicals and radiation sources
- Some medications (check your script with your doctor)
- Recreationally used stimulants, psychoactive drugs and relaxants
- Frequent travel
- Irregular sleep cycles.

So before thinking supplements, think simple lifestyle changes. You can work them out from the above list for yourself. And while you may not be able to change some of these factors, there is adequate reason to perfect those in your control. For a start:

- ✦ Seek the sun early in the morning and have regular doses of the sun throughout the day (artificial lights don't help). Remember, your eyes are the gateway to a healthy pineal gland, not the skin. You do not need to risk sunburn.
- ✦ Achieve effective time management that allows you to be active during the day, and not carry work over into the evening.
- ✦ Do not overwork. Slow down with the sun where possible.
- ✦ Avoid shift work where possible.
- ✦ Match your weekend hours to your work hours, and overall, to sensible sleep cycles.
- ✦ Create a dark sleep environment. Candle and firelight are acceptable but any artificial light is not.
- ✦ Exercise where possible during the day.
- ✦ Minimise time zone travel.
- ✦ Reduce exposure to smoking, alcohol, recreational drugs, pollutants, EMF and any other nasty you can think of.
- ✦ Minimise stress.
- ✦ Finally, follow Sleep Health Principles.

Otherwise, try supplementing as for serotonin. Consider additional antioxidants which support melatonin in its role. Maintain a Healthy Eating Plan.

But as usual, start with simple lifestyle changes first, because your Mindbody is built to cope with life, as long as you don't abuse it.

Treatment of Mild Psychological Disorders

As is clear from the preceding text, our human brain hormones are seriously more complex than our human brains can actually imagine.

For this reason, we strongly advise consultation with a professional in regards to balancing these neurotransmitters rather than trying to treat yourself, particularly if you have major depression or any other diagnosable mental health condition.

Also, while the focus of this section is purely on nutritional medicine, this does not mean that other therapies such as homeopathy, herbs, reflexology, acupuncture, hypnotherapy, Bowen therapy, Body harmony, massage, Bush flower and Bach Flower essences, to name just a few, should be ignored. Each person needs to assess for themselves which particular treatments they are suited to. The important thing is not to be judgemental. Remember, each to their own. Just decide which works for you and leave the rest so others may find what's right for them. In fact we encourage you to try as many approaches as feasible in order to find a solution to your health concerns.

One thing that needs to be said is the importance of personal expression in maintaining psychological health. If we hold onto things, then we slow our healing.

It is obvious now just how much an effect our thoughts and feelings (and the neurotransmitters they subsequently create) have on our body's health and wellbeing. All the vitamins and minerals in the world are not going to help you if you remain in a state of unexpressed, or worse still, negatively expressed living. That is why our first call in this book was 'Be Happy'. Enjoy the Pleasure Principle, the Passion Principle, getting your relationships as perfect as you can and your emotions and reasons under an adequate level of control.

People express in so many different ways, through talking, through art, through running, to name just a few.

The important thing is that you need to express your emotions, whatever method you choose.

If you need help doing this, then find someone who can help you. The sooner you do so, the better you will feel. It's that simple.

This said, the following are some of the nutrients, herbs and amino acids that may help in the treatment of mild psychological disorders. We advise that any supplement regime for mental health should be under the supervision of a practitioner.

NEUROTRANSMITTER HEALTH

Omega 3 fish oils	EPA/DHA 3–9g
Vitamin B6	50–250mg
B Complex	
Zinc (elemental)	35–50mg at bedtime

Magnesium (elemental)	500mg at bedtime
Multivitamin	

FOR DEPRESSION (AS ABOVE PLUS)

St John's Wort	as directed
OR Tryptophan	200–400mg
OR SAMe	400–800mg
OR Tyrosine	500–1000mg

FOR ANXIETY (AS FOR NEUROTRANSMITTER HEALTH PLUS)

Taurine	500–1000mg
OR Inositol	500–1500mg
OR Tyrosine	500–1000mg
OR Glutamine	500–1000mg

Important Notes

+ Never take Tryptophan, SAMe or St John's Wort without medical supervision if you are taking a prescription medication for a psychological disorder.

+ Remember that St John's Wort interacts with so many other prescription medications, including the oral contraceptive pill. Ask your GP or pharmacist to check.

+ Do not take all of the above treatments at once. Either choose Tryptophan, SAMe or St John's Wort. Take the maximum dose as directed for three months to reach maximum effect. Even an anti-depressant drug can take three weeks to have an effect, so allow yourself patience and time.

+ Don't forget foods can have dramatic effect on our moods, as can low levels of blood sugar that is associated with eating irregular meals.

9

Bones, Joints and Muscles

Advice on bone health found in this chapter is particularly pertinent if:

You have a family history of osteoporosis	**Yes / No**
You are female, particularly if approaching or past menopause	**Yes / No**
You have a history of multiple fractures	**Yes / No**
You experience bone pains	**Yes / No**
You have been a heavy smoker or alcohol user	**Yes / No**
You have or have had an eating disorder	**Yes / No**
You have been immobile for a considerable period	**Yes / No**
Particularly if any of the above occurred in your teenage years	**Yes / No**

Advice on joint health found in this chapter is particularly pertinent if:

You have difficulty moving any of your joints	**Yes / No**
You have red or hot joints	**Yes / No**
You have painful joints	**Yes / No**
You have a history of trauma near or to a joint or joints	**Yes / No**

Advice on muscle health found in this chapter is particularly pertinent if:

You experience regular cramps or muscle spasms	**Yes / No**
You suffer from regular aches and pains in the muscles	**Yes / No**
You frequently experience muscular fatigue	**Yes / No**

You have restless leg syndrome	**Yes / No**
You experience muscular tension after stress	**Yes / No**
You have multiple muscles with trigger points	**Yes / No**

Diagnosable diseases specifically involving bone, joint or muscle dysfunction include:

+ Osteoporosis and Osteopaenia, Paget's Disease
+ Osteoarthritis, Rheumatoid Arthritis, Ankylosing Spondylitis and other forms of arthritis
+ Degenerative Vertebral Discs
+ Traumatic Fractures and Sporting Injuries
+ Fibromyalgia, Myofascial Trigger Points
+ Tension Headaches, Neck Pain, Lower Back Pain
+ Anxiety related muscle tension.

Osteopaenia and Osteoporosis

Contrary to what you may believe, the human skeleton is not simply in existence to hang the rest of your body off like a complicated coat hanger. The human skeleton is in fact alive, and an active system that not only supports the body, but acts as a storage system for various minerals. It is not only a hard mix of calcium and phosphate, but contains a blood supply, a protein matrix, and many different minerals essential to its overall health. Ignore this fact at your peril, particularly if you are female, for the consequences of a weak skeletal system may cost you not only your quality of life in your elder years, but through complications of fractures, your life itself.

What does a healthy bone look like? On the surface bone has a hard, enamel like coat, but is like a block of honeycomb within, porous and weblike. What happens when problems with your bones occur? More air than bone appears within the honeycomb-like matrix. This is known as osteopaenia when mild, or osteoporosis when moderate or worse. We have previously discussed relevant tests for this in Chapter 7 of this section, 'Hormone Health'.

What are the consequences of weak bones? Basically, bones that are more likely to fracture when placed under strain.

Who is most vulnerable? Women after menopause, especially who have a history of hormonal imbalance and, in particular, who have had a hysterectomy and oopherectomy without appropriate hormone replacement. Other risk factors include family history, poor dietary habits, lack of weight bearing exercise, eating disorders, smoking and heavy alcohol use. Especially if such a history existed during the adolescent years as this is an important time in determining the ultimate long-term strength of our bones.

So what do you do if you find out you have osteopaenia or osteoporosis? Well, you have already made a start if you are on the Healthy Eating Plan, for you will be:

- Eating a diet both high and in balance with the nutrients required to prevent osteoporosis. These include calcium, magnesium, boron (ensure you are eating nuts and seeds), zinc, magnesium, B group vitamins, manganese and Vitamin K (lots of leafy greens). Your diet will have adequate fibre, a moderate protein intake, high fruit and vegetable intake, a moderate caffeine and alcohol intake (high intake affects bones), healthy fat intake and low sugar intake.
- You should be doing weight bearing exercises. It's as simple as walking. In order to prevent upper limb osteoporosis, add cuff weights to your wrists. Alternatively do 2 or 3 sessions of weighted upper limb exercise in addition to walking per week.
- Don't stress! The stress response pulls magnesium and calcium from your bones in order to aid muscle function during physical crises meaning that long-term stress can affect bone strength.
- Ensure you have a healthy gut. Poor digestion limits mineral intake necessary for bone strength.
- Talk to a nutritionally orientated doctor about the possibility of using natural hormone replacement as an adjunct to the above approaches if required.

✦ Alternatively, there are drugs available to help with bones but these are usually only available once osteoporosis is underway.

And what about supplements? They help, but once again consider the need for a balanced supplement rather than a single megadose. We have already discussed this, and how it is particularly pertinent for osteoporosis. Prevention is not just about calcium, otherwise increasing dairy products would work for all. And it does not. First and foremost, you need to make sure your parathyroid gland is secreting parathyroid hormone in order for a balanced bone matrix to be formed. So before mega-dosing with calcium, think magnesium and B Group Vitamins to get this gland working, after which you can add your calcium.

A good balance is twice as much calcium as magnesium, mixed in with a variety of micro-minerals in lesser but equally important doses; zinc (with a 10:1 ratio of copper), manganese and Vitamin K as well. Get it right and you won't have to megadose.

OSTEOPOROSIS/OSTEOPAENIA (IN ASSOCIATION WITH DIET)

2:1 Ratio of Calcium (1000mg) to Magnesium (500mg)
10:1 Ratio of Zinc (20mg) to Copper(2mg)
Manganese	5 mg
B Complex	
Vitamin K	5 ug
Boron	1–3mg

Osteoarthritis

Osteoarthritis, the 'wear and tear' of your joints and bones, is another common musculoskeletal disorder. Any joint may be affected, but it is usually the hips and knees that limit people most. Simply put, the soft tissue that lines the bone around the joints is slowly degraded leaving less than perfect joint surfaces.

This leaves you with aches and pains about the joint in question. You should be able to differentiate for yourself whether a pain is in the joint or muscle most of the time, but your doctor may be able to clarify the situation with an X-ray if necessary.

What do you do if you suspect osteoarthritis? A good start is to see a physiotherapist, chiropractor, osteopath or exercise therapist who can provide you with guidance, and a carefully considered exercise program. The more strength you have around a joint, the less you will suffer from this condition as long as your exercise program is constructed with respect to any dysfunction that may be occurring. In the latter case a trained eye may be necessary, for it may be your movement patterns that are causing your pain in the first place, and an incorrectly performed exercise program may only make this worse.

The key is not just to exercise, but to exercise right.

This is an area where a good supplement program can also indisputably help. As long as you have only mild or moderate arthritis in which the cartilage forming cells remain intact, there is a solution. Feed them. What do you feed them? They hunger for bonded chains of sugars, proteins and sulphur called glucosamine and chondroitin. The functions of these two formulae overlap as they both help to form the backbone of your cartilage. They are the mesh that binds your cartilage together, while also allowing fluid to sit within like a sponge. The less cartilage matrix you have, the less spongy your cartilage and the more damage done to your joint under the pressure of weight bearing.

Multiple studies show the effectiveness of glucosamine and chondroitin in halting the decline and even rebuilding cartilage damage. No drug will do this. In fact, some commonly used prescription drugs do the reverse, while masking the symptoms of continuing osteoarthritic decline.

Glucosamine and chondroitin come in many shapes and forms. Discuss which formula best suits you with your pharmacist or health food practitioner. Differences include whether it comes in tablet, powdered or oil form. Choose your preference, but realise the powder may come with additional calories due to the high sugar content of the stabilisers used. Another difference is the chemical to which the glucosamine is bound (sulphate, acetate or hydrochloride). Various arguments exist for each, but one compelling reason to choose sulphate formulas is that joints are made from, among other constituents, sulphur, so you are getting additional nutrients from the package.

As for packages, there are 101 different varieties of nutrient combinations that come with glucosamine. A few useful additions include Methylsulfonylmethane (MSM) (an anti-inflammatory sulphur protein), Cetylmyristoleate (CM) (a natural oil lubricant for joints), antioxidant vitamins A, C and E and selenium, manganese (which helps activate glucosamine), calcium orotate and B Group Vitamins. Blends with anti-inflammatory herbs (Bromelian, Quercetin, Turmeric) also exist as well as fish oil supplements, which may more specifically address inflammatory arthritis such as Rheumatoid Arthritis. As a general rule, the more additional ingredients the better, but obviously cost is an issue.

OSTEOARTHRITIS

Glucosamine	1500mg per day
Chondroitin	750mg per day
MSM	250mg
Cetyl Myristoleate	750mg

With Additional B Complex,
Antioxidant vitamins,
Selenium, Zinc, Manganese and Calcium Orotate

Rheumatoid Arthritis

What about the more complex arthritis that occurs as a result of autoimmune disorders, the most common of which is rheumatoid arthritis? These joint disorders require a more detailed and complex approach since their causes and effects occur throughout the body, not just at a local joint level. Thus a supplemental approach does not only take into account the joint needs for glucosamine and so forth, but also includes support for the gastrointestinal and immune systems (see Chapter 10 of this section, 'Creating a Healthy Immune System', for further explanation).

Thus when addressing Rheumatoid Arthritis you might consider:
1. The use of glucosamine/ chondroitin formulas as discussed for Osteoarthritis for repair of joint damage (see above).
2. The inclusion of anti-inflammatory and immune balancing nutrients such as EPA/ DHA fish oils, zinc, antioxidants and B complex (see Chapter 10, 'Creating a Healthy Immune System').

3. Gastrointestinal repair beginning with probiotics and a Food Elimination Regime (including all red meats). Dairy and gluten intolerance are also possibilities (see Chapter 2 of this section, 'Gastrointestinal Health').

RHEUMATOID ARTHRITIS (AND OTHER INFLAMMATORY ARTHRITIS)

Glucosamine plus other Joint Protection   1500mg
Fish Oils(EPA/DHA)   6-9g
Zinc plus other Immune System Support
Probiotics plus other Gastro-Intestinal Interventions and Support (see relevant sections)
Anti-inflammatory herbs (Bromelin, Quercetin, Turmeric)

Muscular Problems

So what about general aches, pains, cramps and fatigue in the muscles? Here we are not talking about any injury or trauma related condition, for which you should see a doctor or musculoskeletal practitioner for a clear diagnosis. Nor are we considering any situation in which the aches, pain or fatigue is occurring in association with wider symptoms of any kind. Again, where systemic symptoms exist in which generalised aches, pain or fatigue are only a part, seek a diagnosis from a doctor or other practitioner.

But otherwise, what should you do about the aches and pains? A quick lesson in how muscles contract and relax. **Muscles contract under the influence of calcium. They relax under the influence of magnesium**. What else do you usually need when your body requires magnesium? Yes, you now know your nutritional biochemistry, the B Group Vitamins. So here is a simple formula that works often for annoying low grade aches, pains, cramps and fatigue.

MUSCLE ACHES AND PAINS

Magnesium (elemental)   500mg
B Complex
Calcium   1000mg

The above formula may also be helpful in cases of persistent myofascial trigger points and fibromyalgia, carpal tunnel syndrome (with added Vitamin B6, 100–200mg), and in aiding recovery from lower back pain, nerve impingement and headaches including migraine.

As for chronic pain, we're now getting complicated as this represents a multifaceted disease process taking in physical, biochemical, mental, emotional and social aspects. But it is worth giving a few additional supplements a try above and beyond what has been recommended. Enter another important neurochemical system, the neuropeptides, endorphins and encephalins. These are our natural wonder drugs when it comes to pain. What are they derived from? The amino acid, phenylalanine. This helps to increase our endorphin levels (so may tyrosine, as it is closely related to phenylalanine). Vitamin E may also be considered here. And if depression concurrently exists with chronic pain, also consider the full range of neurotransmitter support (see Chapter 8 of this section, 'Neurotransmitter Health'), particularly Tryptophan and S-adenyl-methionine (SAMe), which in particular are known to help with chronic pain.

ADDITIONAL CHRONIC PAIN SUPPORT

Phenylalanine	500–1000mg
Vitamin E	500 IU

Plus Neurotransmitter Support if concurrent Depression exists (particularly Tryptophan, SAMe)

The best advice is to try the maximum dose of any of these formulae for a minimum of two months and see how you go. You may notice quick changes with magnesium supplementation, but two-three months is the time frame it may take for other supplementation such as glucosamine to reach full effect (unless topically applied). If the supplements work, slowly reduce the dose and see if you can do without them. If you can't do without supplements, stop at a dosage that maintains your wellbeing (see Section 6, Phase 5, 'Weaning Supplementation'). Of course, if there is no change at all after six-eight weeks, it's not working. Therefore seek further advice.

10

Creating a Healthy Immune System

Information pertaining to general immune support is particularly relevant to you if:

You frequently experience coughs, colds and flus	Yes / No
You frequently get ear, nose or throat infections	Yes / No
You suffer from skin infections such as cold sores	Yes / No
Cuts and wounds are slow to heal	Yes / No

Advice for regulating your immune response in circumstances of hyperimmunity or autoimmune disorder are pertinent to you if:

Your skin and eyes are frequently itchy, dry, light sensitive or irritated	Yes / No
You experience post nasal drip	Yes / No
You experience red, hot swollen joints	Yes / No
You have dark circles beneath your eyes	Yes / No

Diagnosable diseases specifically involving immune system hyperactivity or autoimmunity include:

- Asthma, Hayfever, Sinusitus
- Rheumatoid Arthritis, Ankylosing Spondylitis
- Psoriasis, Eczema
- Scleroderma, Systemic Lupus Erythematosis, Sjrogrens Syndrome
- Hashimoto's and Graves' Disease
- Multiple Sclerosis

Your immune system is your body's defence against invasion. Break the skin, consume a toxin or parasite, breathe in the same, and your immune system should be prepared to protect you from the consequences. In truth it is a system that has been lurking in the background of all our discussions, for the immune system pervades all other systems, and is therefore inextricably linked to each and every other body mechanism.

Experience hormonal imbalance, consume the wrong food, punish the lungs with a cigarette, develop high cholesterol, get too little or indeed too much exercise or simply eat a sugar rich, fat rich, essential fatty acid imbalanced diet, and each and every one of these factors will significantly alter the state of your immune system.

Here is a brief overview of how this system works. First of all your immune system has a general response to tissue injury; be it trauma, temperature, infection, toxin or otherwise caused. This response is known as your 'innate immunity', the general background response available from birth that generates an immediate response to any threat.

As body tissue is injured, histamine and other messengers are released from the damaged area initiating the inflammatory response, in which surrounding blood vessels become porous and hence leak fluid into the area of damage. This in effect is what you see as swelling when you sprain an ankle, but it happens with any insult to the body. Along with the fluid arrive white blood cells and clotting factors, to seal any damaged blood vessels.

A host of white blood cells with names such as macrophages, neutrophils, eosinophils and so forth arrive to 'phagocytose' the cell. This in effect means they surround the damaged tissue or invading toxin or parasite, and gobble it up. Those of you who remember the video game 'Pacman' will understand the concept. Each of the different white blood cells has a different role, so they all need to be healthy for you to be healthy.

So how do we make them healthy? You might have guessed the answer already. They are cells. So give them Cellular Health. Furthermore, these are cells attacking damaged tissues and micro-organisms, and hence need to combat released toxins. So they will need to be particularly healthy in their role of preventing free radical damage as a consequence of the oxidation of debris. Think antioxidants. And they'll need lots of energy too, so B Group Vitamins are also in order. Now they of course have their own specific requirements but here is where it gets complicated so we'll not go into the details as to why. We will simply tell you, more than anything, they like Vitamin C and the anti-inflammatory components found in garlic. Other herbs that aid the innate immune response include ginger, quercetin (found in onion), boswelia and turmeric.

So here's a suggestion when your immunity is down. Have a lot of fresh ginger, garlic, turmeric, fresh onion, and vegetables (green peppers are high in Vitamin C); try an Asian stir-fry or salad with lots of greens rather than rice or noodles (light on the oil) or a laksa soup. Traditional homemade stock soups are also filled with nutrients to assist you in this process. Keep the sugars in your diet light as they feed any bug you are hosting, so do not overdo the fruits in your quest for Vitamin C. A host of coloured vegetables will do, adding to your all-round nutrient load.

Or, of course, you can always supplement.

GENERAL IMMUNE SYSTEM SUPPORT

Vitamin C	At least 3g daily
Garlic	3–18g daily
Zinc	35–50mg elemental bedtime

With additional High Strength Antioxidant Support daily including

Vitamin A	3500 IU
Vitamin E	250–500 IU
Selenium	150ug

(see Chapter 1 'Cellular Health' for more details)

Additional herbal support from Ginger, Boswellia and Turmeric, Quercetin as directed on bottle.

Please note that your body will tell you when you have absorbed enough Vitamin C as you will experience diarrhoea. So for the short-term, don't be afraid to take enough Vitamin C to allow this to happen, then slowly reduce your dose as your deficiency dwindles.

And don't forget a source of omega-3 fats. The essential fatty acids are critical in the inflammatory response. Not so much in making it happen as ensuring that the inflammatory response does not go too far and overshoot into chronic inflammation. Put simply, this has to do with how aggressively your body responds to inflammation. There are various messengers the body uses to understand its own state of inflammation with complicated names yet again (prostaglandins, leukotrienes, thromboxanes and so forth). Each has a part to play in the body's response; some encourage the continuation of inflammation and others help mediate and turn off the response when appropriate.

Here's the catch. The pro-inflammatory mediators, those that prolong inflammation, are built from omega-6 fatty acids, those you predominantly get from meat and vegetable oils. The inflammation controlling mediators, those that slow down and stop inflammation when it is no longer necessary, are built from Omega-3 fatty acids, those you get from deep water fish.

So what happens when you don't get enough fish oils due to a dietary imbalance? You run the risk of continued inflammation when it is no longer necessary, since you are creating more pro-inflammatory mediators than anti-inflammatory ones. Result? Chronic swelling and a continued inflammatory response well past its use-by date. Outcome? A worsening outcome on almost all chronic diseases and even obesity.

This gets complicated so we will leave our explanation with a simple example. Cholesterol circulating about the body is normal. This is how we distribute the building blocks for our sex hormones, amongst other things. But a pro-inflammatory environment creates problems, particularly if we also lack antioxidants to neutralise the oxidant risk associated with cholesterol. For once denatured by free radicals (if not protected by antioxidants), cholesterol will be zealously set upon by our own immune system.

The result? Atherosclerotic plaque from oxidised cholesterol deposits then build up in our blood vessel walls under the continued attack of our immune system. This, in effect, narrows the arteries leading to eventual occlusion, with the added risk that a chunk of plaque may break off and plug up an artery downstream. The outcome, angina or heart attack. Or if the plug is in the brain, a stroke.

This is one reason why we need to control our immune system by consuming fish, or supplementing with fish oils.

| Omega-3 Fish Oils | EPA/DHA | 4–9g |

Of course, given that the insult to your body may have a specific cause such as trauma or infection, it also pays to address the intruder in question. Physical damage is the most easy to identify, but your body should be well capable of supplying adequate nutrients to deal with this situation from your diet in most cases, unless the trauma is significant, in which case you should be under the care of a professional anyway.

But what about infections? Coughs and colds, stomach upsets (make sure you've read Chapter 2 of this section, 'Gastrointestinal Health'), urinary tract infections, thrush and the like. Well, what you can do to specifically address an infection will depend upon what the infection is caused by. Is it a virus (a partial organism that invades your cell to reproduce), a bacteria or fungus (a small single cell or multicellular organism) or a parasite (a larger organism)? There are natural herbal remedies for each, but what works for one may not work for another, and ultimately, depending upon the organism, a prescription drug (antibiotic, antifungal etc) followed by probiotic rehabilitation may be a better option.

Given that herbal remedies for each are generally without side effects and are not expensive, you could try a 'blind' attempt at treatment over a one to two week period, but if symptoms persist or are serious, seek a better idea of what is causing your particular symptoms through diagnostic testing. General herbs to consider include echinacea (used as a specific treatment, preferably not on an ongoing basis), astragalus membranaceus (particularly for upper respiratory tract infections), berberine, boswellia, ginger, oregano oil, olive leaf extract or artemisia.

There are one or two specific clues to guide your treatment. In the case of urinary tract infections, consider cranberry, either as 100 per cent juice (no sugar added) or as an extract in capsule form. Do not use sweetened juice for you'll be feeding the bacteria sugar and helping it multiply at the same time that you are trying to kill it, complicating the battle.

FOR PREVENTION OF URINARY TRACT INFECTIONS

100 per cent Cranberry Juice (unsweetened)
Cranberry Capsules (17,000mg)1-2/day

Please note that cranberry works primarily as a preventative against UTI's. In our experience, we have found cranberry can effectively mask symptoms of UTI's but not actually treat the underlying infection, as shown by urine cultures presumably post-infection. So be careful here. Generally one to two capsules are enough for prevention. In the short-term this can be increased to six capsules per day.

For coughs and throat infections (assuming it is not a lung infection), use a zinc lozenge (suck, don't swallow). Echinacea and astragalus are also helpful here. But remember your high dose garlic and Vitamin C as well.

COUGHS AND THROAT INFECTIONS

Zinc lozenges	35–50mg elemental
Garlic	3–18 grams, short term
Vitamin C	To bowel tolerance
Echinacea (short-term)	As directed
Astragalus	As directed

Cold sores (the herpes simplex virus) are stimulated by a high intake of the amino acid arginine (good for erections and sperm fertility, bad for herpes, now that's nature at its cruellest!) and high stress levels. So stop arguing with your partner, then emotionally eating chocolates and nuts (high arginine foods), and making up afterwards (rubbing vulnerable tissues). Instead, take lysine, Vitamin C and use zinc lozenges once again.

COLD SORES/ HERPES

Lysine	3g (500mg–1g preventative dosage)
Vitamin C	3g
Zinc Lozenges	35–50mg elemental

And while we are at it, we might just need to tread a little water in the controversial area of Candida. Alternately blamed for everything and argued not to exist, let's confine our discussion to the irrefutable oral or vaginal thrush. You can read in great detail elsewhere whether or not it is causing you any number of systemic problems; from mental health to vagueness, faltering immunity to reproductive system imbalance, fatigue to flatulence, obesity and weight gain.

Over the last decade in particular these wide ranging symptoms have also been blamed on Insulin Resistance, Thyroid Imbalance, Adrenal Crisis,

Leaky Gut, Toxic Liver and any number of latest trend explanations whose symptoms seem to cover all conditions. This is not to say that all of the above are not potentially a candidate for causing each of these problems and in turn each other. However, you really need to know what it is that is causing **YOUR** problem. If your symptoms are widespread, you should be seeing a professional to clarify the situation, or at least to clarify what is of priority among a hierarchy of conditions, in treating **YOUR** systemic condition.

In any case, back to oral or vaginal thrush, and in particular, systemic Candida. Here's what you can do. Please note that this regime must continue for two to three months if any effect is to be achieved. It involves a very restrictive diet, and nutrition supplementation is absolutely essential for this regime.

There are three ways to eliminate an excess of Candida and all three must be performed simultaneously:

1. You must starve the Candida by restricting those foods that it feeds on.
2. You must actively kill the Candida by supplementing with both natural herbs, and, ideally, antifungal drugs.
3. You must replenish your good gut bacteria (probiotics).

There are many books now available that focus solely on the elimination of Candida from the body. Candida recipe books also abound. Although there may be subtle differences, most diet plans are very similar.

- You must restrict yourself to completely natural and fresh foods (no processed or canned foods).
- You must eliminate all natural 'yeast' foods from your diet. These include mushrooms, vinegar, nuts, olives, pickles and beer. You must also exclude wheat products, oats, sugar, fermented foods, chilli peppers, peppers, eggplant, alcohol and dairy.
- For the first month, all fruits must be excluded as they are high in sugar, after which restrict to small amounts only during the second month.

INVESTIGATING YOUR PERSONAL SUPPLEMENT NEEDS

As stated previously, nutritional supplementation is essential. There are many varied regimes, but the following regime is very successful in the vast majority of compliant individuals.

CANDIDA (FOR 2 MONTHS)

Probiotics	1–2 capsules before breakfast
Garlic	3g twice daily
Olive Leaf Extract	
Artemesia, Black Walnut, Citrus Seed Extract	Maximum directed dose

Some stronger compounds such as caprylic acid with molybdenum (available from compounding chemists) may also be necessary.

In our experience, the addition of two weeks of antifungal drugs (Nystatin) at the very beginning of the regime greatly increases your chances of being successful. This is only available on prescription from your doctor.

Nystatin	(500,000 IU)	2 tablets, 3 times daily

There are two more points to make here. On starting this regime, it is quite common to feel worse (sometimes significantly worse) before you feel better. This is due to the toxic by-products that are formed when Candida dies. Usually this period is over within a week, buut sometimes it can be prolonged. If you can get through this, you are doing your Mindbody a world of good. Despite the seeming contradiction, sometimes it may be necessary to take some paracetamol, for example, for you to continue with the journey. Do not berate yourself for this; medication has its place. Just remember, it is often the case that the worse you feel at the beginning, the more likely it is that you are following the correct path to your own personal health.

Another important gem is that sometimes excess Candida will simply not go away. In such cases there may be other underlying conditions, such as a burden of heavy metals (such as mercury) within your body. Treat the underlying condition and the Candida should disappear. As easy as this program sounds, we recommend you seek professional assistance as this may be quite a long and cumbersome journey.

At the end of your two months, you may stop all supplements other than the probiotics. These should be maintained for at least six months. Now, we recommend you follow the principles of Food Reintroduction found in Chapter 7 (Food Elimination Regime). Yes, this does extend your restricted dietary time further, but it does allow you to be truly aware of which foods in particular may be toxic to you.

So we have your immune system covered. Or do we? Actually, we have only covered the simple part. We have yet to discuss your acquired immune system, that part of your immune system that remembers past insults and reacts accordingly when they are repeated. To keep things simple, we will not go into 'how it works'. Rather we will spend more time on what happens when it doesn't work effectively.

After an invasion by a foreign body (virus, bacteria, fungus, parasite), the immune system produces a memory of the invader via the creation of antibodies. These antibodies are then able to quickly latch onto a repeat invasion of a foreign body so as to mount a more effective defence. The phagocytic cells previously discussed are more effectively able to attack and break down the foreign body as a result of the antibody's contribution to the acquired immune system function.

This is a very effective system when the antibody defence system is accurately able to establish between Self and invader, but trouble arises when the immune system makes mistakes. Either the system becomes hyperreactive against those foreign bodies to which it is repeatedly exposed or, worse still, the immune system starts to attack its own body as if it were a foreign invader itself.

The result is what is known as Hyperreactive Inflammatory Diseases such as sinusitis, hayfever, asthma and inflammatory bowel disease (Crohn's and ulcerative colitis) or Autoimmune diseases, which include such conditions as rheumatoid arthritis, ankylosing spondylitis, psoriasis, systemic lupus erythematosis and multiple sclerosis.

This is an area where dysfunction can become disease. It is vitally important to indicate here the need to identify root causes in order to down-regulate the inflammatory state. Nutrients to address these complicated conditions must comprise of:

1. A combination of vitamins, minerals and essential fatty acids to both address balancing the immune system and inflammatory response.
2. A supply of key nutrients to assist the function of the areas set upon by the condition with an attempt to repair the damage already done.

A preceding step to both these interventions is to **establish the health of the gut first, whether the condition is in the gut or elsewhere.** For if the gut is leaking large food particles or micro-organisms about the body, these foreign invaders will to be lodged elsewhere, be it in the joints, the skin or even the brain, resulting in possible hyperreactive or autoimmune system responses, as we often see in cases of rheumatoid arthritis, psoriasis, psoriatic arthritis and eczema, to name a few.

Although this might not have seemed logical before the beginning of this book, we hope by now it makes simple sense. Particularly consider:

1. A course of probiotics
2. A Food Elimination Regime
3. Repair of Leaky Gut Syndrome.

Following the Food Elimination Regime, a Healthy Eating Plan is a must. The above conditions represent one situation where a significant reduction in all types of red meat may be especially helpful. Trial a reduction in red meat (especially servings containing high fat) or even cessation of eating red meat for six weeks to establish if it contributes to your hyperreactive inflammatory or autoimmune state (add it to your Food Elimination Regime).

Your body will advise you what to do next. It may be necessary to stay off red meat for an extended period of time. If this is the case, maintain your protein levels with a quality protein powder. Vitamin B6, B12 and zinc may also need protective supplementing in this case, as well as iron, although the latter only in the low dosages previously suggested (35mg or less), as it may lead to pro-inflammatory states if overdone.

So in summary, a comprehensive approach to these conditions should address:

1. Gastrointestinal Health
2. Immune System Health
3. The health of the particular system or systems involved

Consultation with a specialist is likely to be necessary in most of these conditions.

11

Vision, Hearing and Headaches

If you have any concerns regarding your vision or hearing, you should be reviewed by your doctor, optometrist, ophthalmologist or audiologist first. After which, the following chapter provides information regarding the protection of eye and ear health.

The eyes require a balanced nutrient intake if they are to remain a finely tuned sensory organ. Not only are they sensitive to nutritional intake, they are also vulnerable to systemic imbalances such as blood sugar irregularities and high blood pressure. Thus they need particular attention if they are to remain in healthy and finetuned condition, particularly as we age.

An obvious area of concern for the eyes is the effect of light upon their health. Excessive light exposure leads to oxidation of any external area of the body, but the eyes are particularly vulnerable. Thus the Antioxidant Nutrients such as Vitamin A (in particular), C and E, as well as zinc, selenium, lipoic acid, bioflavonoids and the carotenoids (lutein) are very important.

As with all cells, the more complicated line of toxin defence involving the antioxidant enzymes (superoxide dismutase and glutathione based enzymes) also assists in this process thus indicating a possible place for supplementation with glutamine and other associated amino acids, methionine, cysteine and glycine. Re-read Chapter 1 of this section, 'Cellular Health', for a revision if necessary.

The B Group vitamins including folate also play a part in healthy eye maintenance, as will Omega-3 fats where inflammation is involved. Many of the above are now available in composite eye formulas for ease of supplementation.

Of course, protecting your eyes first is the best line of defence. Here you should always consider:

- Having your eyes checked regularly for declining vision
- Wearing sunglasses
- Quitting smoking, or avoid smoky environments
- Breaking up long periods of computer use or reading
- Ensuring adequate lighting is available
- Eating healthy foods that will provide you with a comprehensive range of nutrients from different food groups. Remember those carrots and a multitude of other fruit and vegetables!

A further consideration is controlling any systemic condition that may affect the eyes. This includes:

- Insulin Resistance or Diabetes, which can lead to Diabetic Retinopathy
- High Blood Pressure
- Food and Chemical Intolerances

There are also herbs that may assist in the health of the eyes, one of which is bilberry. The other important consideration is the avoidance of vegetable oils, which have recently been shown to contribute to macular degeneration.

EYE HEALTH

Broad based Antioxidant
Magnesium and B Complex
Omega-3 Fish Oils   EPA/DHA   4g
Bilberry   1–3g dried fruit
Lutein   5–30mg

As for optimal eyesight, antioxidants and B Group vitamins are again critical in hearing loss. However, an added consideration is supplementation with Vitamin D and calcium, as per supplementation for osteoporosis (see Chapter 9 of this section, 'Bones, Joints and Muscles') as hearing is dependent upon sound translation through the small bones of the ears.

Headaches

Headaches are generally caused by one of five possibilities.

1. **Dehydration**—The most common cause. Make sure you are drinking 1.5–2 litres of water per day.
2. **Neck problems**—Once again, high dose magnesium may help with any neck stiffness, muscle tightness or spasm that may be contributing to headache. A 'hands on' therapist such as a physiotherapist, chiropractor, osteopath or myofascial therapist may also be required here to assist with both diagnosis and treatment.
3. **Deteriorating eyesight**—As stated above, always get your eyes thoroughly checked before embarking on a full headache regime.
4. **Hormonal imbalances**—Headaches of this type most commonly occur in pre- or perimenopausal women. The most common time is before menstruation; however, such headaches can occur at any time in the cycle. Most women know when there is a hormonal component to their headaches. Please see Chapter 7 of this section, 'Hormone Health', for information regarding treatment as hormonal headaches are most commonly due to progesterone deficiency.
5. **Food intolerances**—Red wine, cheese, oranges and chocolate are well accepted as potential triggers for migraine. However, any food can cause a headache as a result of food intolerance if you are susceptible. By now, you would be aware of any food intolerances by having undergone the Food Elimination Regime.

Of course, there are other more serious causes of headaches such as acoustic neuromas and brain tumours. If the above measures do not result in an improvement in your headaches, then it is time to be assessed by your doctor.

12

Skin, Nails and Hair

The following chapter is pertinent if:

You have a particular interest in your cosmetic appearance	**Yes / No**
You have particular problems with your skin (acne, psoriasis, eczema)	**Yes / No**
You have poor nail or hair quality	**Yes / No**

Your personal appearance may or may not be of great concern to you. But the appearance of your skin, lips and tongue, as well as your eyes and hair, is often a helpful indication in reading the balance of nutrients in your system. In this sense, treating your appearance can often in turn have beneficial effects on your health.

Take the simple case of pimples, more technically known as acne. Other than family history, what contributes to acne?

- Food intolerances
- Stress including heat, exercise, mechanical trauma
- Insulin Resistance; excess sugars in your system exacerbate acne
- Hormonal Imbalances; explaining adolescent acne occurrence
- High saturated fat diets
- Facial products; inappropriate soaps, creams and cosmetics.

Now, we have already talked about combating all of the above previously **IF** implicated. After which, there are specific nutrients that are of most benefit to skin. Again, Healthy Lifestyle first, including moderate exercise and an Healthy Eating Plan. Then consider nutrient assistance, if necessary. Which nutrients are good for the skin in particular?

SKIN HEALTH

EPA/DHA	4–6g
Zinc (elemental)	35–50mg bedtime
Probiotics	2 capsules before breakfast

Vitamins A (as Betacarotene), C & E, B Complex including B5 (Pantothenic Acid), B6, Biotin, Manganese
Vitamin D3 may also be necessary for psoriasis 2-4000IU

It is important to note, however, that, unlike most nutritional regimes, six months rather than three seems to be necessary for adequate treatment if skin conditions exist.

Yet the vital question to ask is this. What is more important to treat; Insulin Resistance, Hormonal Imbalance or Acne? Therefore, if there is a limit to the supplements or other measures you want to take, we recommend you seriously prioritise your concerns (i.e. Insulin Resistance or Hormonal Imbalance), and see if other lesser issues (i.e. skin conditions) subsequently go away as well.

A short note on the more complex skin conditions such as psoriasis and eczema. These diseases often represent complex disorders involving the skin, immune and, in some instances, gastrointestinal systems, as well as environmental influences. Thus more complex combined health interventions are appropriate which include:

1. The first place to begin is to review the use of any topically applied soaps, lotions or other products, and avoid airborne toxins such as cigarette smoke. Seek natural alternatives (check the label to make sure they are as natural as possible).
2. Treat the skin supplementing with antioxidants (Vitamins A, C, E, selenium, lipoic acid), anti-inflammatory nutrients (zinc, B Complex) including EPA/ DHA fish oils (see above).
3. A definite place here for treating the gut with probiotics and a Food Elimination Regime (wheat, dairy and sugars are often implicated).
4. Decrease stress as much as possible.

What about the effects of ageing on the skin? Make sure there is a full complement of antioxidants (e.g. additional Vitamin E and selenium) in any supplement you choose as well. And the simplest intervention of all?

Limit your sun exposure during peak UV light periods (middle of the day), while maintaining some sun hours during the morning and late afternoon in order to activate Vitamin D for bone health. Wear protective clothing and a quality sun protection cream on your exposed areas.

Nails and Hair

Your nails can tell you much about the state of several key nutrients. Simply speaking, nice nails, good health. Do you have any white marks on your nails? If so, there is a high likelihood that you have a zinc deficiency. Frequently cracked, brittle and peeling nails? You may need Biotin (with a complete B complex), silica, essential fatty acids, and in some cases, iron (if nails are brittle and ridged). A protein source known as keratin, made up in part by the amino acid cysteine, may also help. However, many other minerals also form the nail bed with less obvious effects on appearance (selenium, sulphur, calcium to name a few), so a good micro-mineral formula may be in order if you are looking for healthy nails.

A good hair formula should be made up of many of the same nutrients as nails. A B complex (including folate) will help take away the dullness, zinc helps bring back the strength, and silicon and keratin provide much of the backbone. Essential fatty acids are also extremely important and their deficiency can be linked to excess dandruff.

As an aside, always make sure the products you use do not contain known carcinogens, a full list of which can be obtained from *The Chemical Maze* by Bill Stratham, a small guidebook on additives and the known risks to your body.

HAIR AND NAIL HEALTH: AS FOR SKIN HEALTH PLUS ...

Silica	20–30mg
Cysteine	500mg
With additional micro-minerals e.g. Sulphur, Selenium	

Lips and Tongue

As with the nails, so with the lips and tongue. A simple guide to many of the B group vitamins is literally on the tip of your tongue.

A deep line down the centre of your tongue? Strawberry in colour? Consider Vitamin B3 deficiency.

Want to know about your folate levels? Is your tongue painful?

Swollen tongue? Consider Vitamin B6.

And purplish or flat, featureless tongue? Consider Vitamin B2 or B12.

Do you want a little confirmation? Here's some lip service.

Cracked corners of the mouth? Vitamins B2, B3 or B12.

If in doubt as to what all this means: simple.

A quality B Complex including folate and added magnesium will cover all of these issues.

LIPS AND TONGUE

B Complex (with Magnesium)
With additional Vitamin B12   500–1000mg

13

Anti-Ageing

Consider this chapter if you are over 45, and have a particular interest in the hyper-health approach advocated by anti-ageing enthusiasts.

In recent years, anti-ageing interventions have been promoted in the name of increasing life longevity and quality. While a Utopian view of age extension is understandable, the view that this will arise simply through the manipulation of particular human biology such as hormones is questionable at best. At least at present, it would appear more appropriate to argue that any interest in age extension should come through optimising health rather than by other means, with increased quality of life arising through a search for continued happiness from this moment onwards rather than the discovery of a dream elixir.

Indeed, most of the factors that appear most likely to extend human years are simply those health factors that prevent the diseases that restrict the quality and quantity of our lives in the first place. Therefore, assuming that you do not presently have a disease, the best approach to increasing the quality and quantity of your years is to enhance the health of those systems that are most vital to your survival.

Is anything more obvious than this?

So if you are healthy and want to prolong your years, what should you focus on? Well, here is our suggestion:

1. Follow the general health principles outlined in the first half of this book directed at maintaining Psychological and Emotional Health. These should include:
    i) Learning to approach life through Acceptance, Humour and Gratitude
    ii) Living with Passion, Pleasure and Optimism

ii) Developing Emotional Intelligence
   iv) Stress Reduction

2. Follow the non-specific health principles directed at maintaining Physical Health:
   i) Cardiovascular Exercise
   ii) Healthy Eating including adequate protein
   iii) Minimisation of Environmental Toxin load
   iv) Sleep Health

There is an additional suggestion pertinent to longevity that should be emphasised and that is **Resistance Training**. Why? Because muscle bulk has been identified as important for providing a reserve of protein to protect against acute illness. In particular, muscle provides a reserve pool for the protein glutamine, which is redistributed about the body during an acute health crisis. You may remember glutamine as the amino acid recommended for healing the gut lining if you have leaky gut. It also may be used for fuelling the immune system, wound healing and other crisis needs.

This highlights the importance of a moderate protein intake as advocated by our Healthy Eating Plan. You cannot build muscles without protein. A diet absent of adequate levels of protein is therefore a diet that does not meet the criteria for health maintenance, and definitely does not fulfil the description of 'Anti-ageing'.

3. Minimise the effects of the diseases that cause the greatest mortality and morbidity in the ageing population. And in turn identify the common risk factors for these diseases
   i) Ceasing Smoking.
   ii) Protecting against Insulin Resistance (basting yourself in high blood sugars and insulin progresses the biological clock considerably).
   iii) Reducing Cholesterol levels.
   iv) Protecting against free radical and oxidation damage through use of antioxidants.

- v) Protecting against methylation errors through control of Homocysteine.
- vi) Down-regulation of the Immune System to prevent Pro-inflammatory states.
- vii) Gut Maintenance and Liver Support to prevent toxic burden on the system.
- viii) Healthy Hormone and Neurotransmitter Balance (sex, adrenal, thyroid, neurotransmitters).
- ix) Supporting the Circulatory System to prevent High Blood Pressure, Anaemia and Clotting Disorders (leading to stroke).
- x) Encouraging Strong Bones to prevent the debilitating and life threatening consequences of fractures as a consequence of falls (particularly but not exclusive to older women).

Now, you should already know how to address these conditions, with or without supplements. The non-specific health interventions already listed incidentally cover the criteria for an anti-ageing regime. As for supplements, it all depends on how much you wish to spend in time, money and emotional input. Don't expect an aggressive argument here from the authors. We believe ageing is a natural aspect of life that should not be tainted by an obsessive fear of decline or desire for life extension.

SECTION 6

Putting It All Together

Most self-help books deal primarily with a single focus, just touching on the occasional side issues. For instance, get the diet right, think a little about exercise, and a long silence on happiness and mental health. As you have noticed, this book is different. After all, you come as a complete package, so why not also your own personal user guide to Health **AND** Happiness?

For this reason, what follows is a Wellbeing Program that relies on creating a Total Health Plan through different intervention stages. While seven phases of health intervention may at first appear complex for this book, it is through respecting these different stages that you will be able to finetune your individual health program according to your own personal needs.

A further advantage of our 7-Phase Program is to give you the flexibility to acclimatise to lifestyle change. Rather than a formal 'kick-start', we'd rather you experience a little tickle into action, followed by a growing momentum of enthusiasm as you actually feel the benefits of change. No scales, but a smile. No self imposed pressures, but a growing realisation that being healthy is the greatest step towards happiness you can make, and being happy, in turn, is the most likely motivation towards positive action and change available!

PHASE 1

Getting Happy!

Time Frame: 3 Weeks

The first phase in your Whole Health Program is to set yourself a stable and firm base for living. One of the most common errors made when people set about creating healthier lives is to pursue a single health aspect without first placing their whole life in perspective. For diet and exercise, the two most common health interventions, along with disease management, will rarely, if ever, bring about happiness of themselves.

Slimmer figures, healthier lives, but if the smile remains absent, how much will you really care? There are a lot of thin, fit, angry, stressed or depressed people out there who are not going to live much longer than many others who are not necessarily the ideal weight, yet are happy and satisfied with who they are.

So to Phase 1: Getting Happy. This phase comprises of three weeks of gradual Self-health involvement. The more eager can 'kick-start' themselves if they like by bypassing this program, but only if you can presently look at yourself with complete honesty and profess,

'I am truly happy and healthy of mind, with few issues of note that will prevent me wholeheartedly committing to my Whole Health Program'.

Can you look at yourself in the mirror and say this?

If not, then Phase 1: Getting Happy, is absolutely essential for your ongoing wellbeing.

WEEK 1:

1. Begin this week with an emphasis on the Pleasure Principle (Section 1, Chapter 3). Getting in touch with your body through simple stretches or a massage would be a good place to start. Whatever your choice, ensure that at least 30 minutes a day are dedicated to pleasing your Self.

2. Increase your levels of activity without yet focusing on structuring an exercise program (next week's concern). Go for a walk. Get back to nature. Enjoy. During these periods investigate your reasoning and motives for improving your health (Section 1, Chapters 4–5).

3. Begin to institute the qualities of Patience, Persistence, Positive Attitude, Personal Achievement, Acceptance and Gratitude into your life (Section 1, Chapter 6). Add a little Humour for good measure (Section 2, Chapter 6). We suggest you purchase a diary or journal during this week, as many surprising and enlightening thoughts may come to mind.

4. Enjoy what is left of the less-than-healthy foods in your pantry. Do not restock your pantry with foods that will not fit into the Healthy Eating Plan outlined in Section 3. If you are going to follow a Food Elimination Regime (we strongly recommend this), do not stock any foods that you will be temporarily removing from your diet.

5. While you may be keen to begin a supplement program, restrict yourself to the following supplements only where specifically indicated:

    i) A good quality probiotic, particularly if you are experiencing gastrointestinal problems (Section 3, Chapter 7). You will need at least 2–3 weeks to review the state of your digestive system.

    ii) A zinc supplement if you have any signs of zinc deficiency.

    iii) A quality B Complex with Magnesium if you lack energy, are experiencing muscular aches, pains or fatigue, or are under considerable stress.

WEEK 2:

1. Review the joys of your week and absorb yourself in the lessons of putting Self First (Section 2, Chapter 1).
2. Investigate your Passions, your Relationships, Emotions and Beliefs (Section 2, Chapters 2–4). You'll therefore have something to think about during the start of your exercise program.
3. Undertake a 30–45 minute walk on at least 5 out of 7 days at a pace you are comfortably challenged by. If you are already undertaking a satisfactory exercise program, you do not have to change it (Section 2, Chapter 7).
4. Review your Sleep Health, and institute any relevant changes indicated (Section 2, Chapter 9).
5. Institute as much of the Healthy Eating Plan as you feel comfortable with. Remember, since you may be undertaking a Food Elimination Regime you **DO NOT** have to institute a full eating plan as yet. However, adapting your eating patterns in sensible ways such as decreasing cereals/grains and increasing fruit and vegetable intake will help you to accommodate either a Healthy Eating Plan or Food Elimination Regime in the coming weeks.

WEEK 3:

1. Continue exercising. If you want to introduce new forms of activity/ exercise, do so slowly.
2. Commit yourself to performing a Relaxation activity on a daily basis (Section 2, Chapter 8).
3. Investigate areas of your life that are stressing you and identify actions that you can undertake in the short and long-term to resolve these issues. Start reading a book on **Time Management** if this is an area of concern for you.
4. During this week, focus on changing the cooking techniques you predominantly use, moving towards salads, soups, stir-frying,

steaming, smoothies and so forth, and away from pan or deep-frying, barbecuing and takeaway meals.

5. For those preparing to undertake a Food Elimination Regime, enjoy a weekend of fine dining and culinary indulgence on quality foods if you wish. Enjoy, because for the next few weeks your diet will be restricted. (Remember, sensible restrictions still apply if you already have dietary limitations as determined by your health status).

A Guide to Phase 1 Supplementation

During the initial phase of your health program we suggest limited supplementation only. This is to ensure that you initially focus on the fundamentals of natural health and happiness as your number one priority. As a consequence, we suggest focusing on only three supplement groups to begin with; probiotics, magnesium (with B Complex) and/or zinc, for these nutrients are vital for the absorption of other nutrients, energy maintenance and healthy digestion.

The following should help you to establish your Phase 1 supplement program:

TAKE A MAGNESIUM SUPPLEMENT (WITH B COMPLEX) IF:

1. You experience eyelid or other body twitches
2. You have heart palpitations, in the absence of known cardiac disease
3. You have restlessness or restless legs
4. You have feelings of tightness or cramps in your legs or feet
5. You experience chocolate cravings, particularly before periods
6. You generally suffer from fatigue

OR IF YOU HAVE ANY OTHER INDICATIONS FOR MAGNESIUM SUPPLEMENTATION IDENTIFED IN SECTION 5.

TAKE A ZINC SUPPLEMENT IF:

1. Food has little taste to you

2. You have white spots on your fingernails indicating zinc deficiency
3. You have poor immunity to coughs, colds or other infections
4. You have slow healing of wounds
5. You are experiencing mouth ulcers or cold sores

OR IF YOU HAVE ANY OTHER INDICATIONS FOR ZINC SUPPLEMENTATION IDENTIFED IN SECTION 5.

TAKE A PROBIOTIC IF YOU EXPERIENCE:
1. Abdominal bloating
2. Abdominal cramps or discomfort
3. Intermittent constipation
4. Intermittent diarrhoea
5. Excess burping
6. Excess flatulence
7. Indigestion

OR IF YOU HAVE ANY OTHER INDICATIONS FOR PROBIOTIC SUPPLEMENTATION IDENTIFED IN SECTION 5.

PHASE 2

Individualising Your Personal Health

Time Frame: 3 Weeks

We all have individual requirements based on our genetic inheritance, state of health and personal preferences. The easiest individual requirement to personally evaluate and manage is your diet. Therefore during Phase 2 of your health plan it is recommended that you undertake a Food Elimination Regime, unless you are absolutely certain you have no digestive concerns. Hopefully you have already followed a two-week probiotic intervention, which may have eradicated some (or all) gastrointestinal symptoms. However, also realise non-gastrointestinal symptoms of Food Intolerances exist, and therefore may also indicate the need for a Food Elimination Regime.

Please remember that this regime also serves as a general detoxification. Many patients in our experience choose to do the Food Elimination Regime even if they have no specific problems entirely for its detoxification value. It is also a wonderful 'kick start' to weight loss for the vast majority of people. Therefore during Phase 2 you should:

1. Undertake the 3 week Elimination Stage of the Elimination Regime if indicated **OR** dedicate yourself to following the Healthy Eating Plan if you believe you have no Food Intolerances. The former option is strongly recommended.
2. Continue all other interventions recommended during Phase 1.
3. Review your life to establish any environmental toxins that you feel comfortable eliminating.

PHASE 3

Addressing Primary Health Dysfunctions

Time Frame: Minimum of 4 Weeks to 3 Months

You are six weeks into your program and it is now time to get down to the business of finetuning your health. But, you might be asking, why haven't you addressed important heath issues earlier?

The reason is that hopefully you will already be feeling much better than when you started this Whole Health Program, without the need for specific supplementation. Why? Because you will have already addressed many of the fundamental principles of healthy living required to ultimately return you towards feeling better. Perhaps not enough to return you to 100 per cent wellbeing, particularly if you have entered this program with a diagnosable disease, but enough improvement to allow you to be more specific in your choice of supplements where required.

For instance, if you have gastrointestinal dysfunction, then the elimination of various foods from your diet combined with a course of probiotics may provide you with significant health gains so that your digestive tract has been returned to a state of wellbeing. Similarly the elimination phase of the regime is such that early weight loss and glycemic control is likely and, in turn, the beginning of cardiovascular health, blood pressure regulation and hormonal balance due to their strong interrelationship with Insulin Resistance.

We are not suggesting that all of a sudden perfect health will have been established. However, you will optimistically have come along enough in your commitment to healthy living to establish how much purely natural life management interventions (diet, exercise, relaxation, emotional intelligence, pleasure, passion and sleep) will assist in overcoming health and happiness dysfunctions. After which it is time to try more direct interventions to address any remaining health conditions, as prioritised by you or your health advocate.

So if you have any identifiable diseases or dysfunctions, what are you going to address first and foremost?

Only you can answer this question. You will need to establish which of the health dysfunctions discussed in Section 5 are most pertinent to you at this point in your life. This may be different to six weeks ago when you first started this program due to improvements established through lifestyle modification. Look through the list of questions at the start of each chapter, as well as the pertinent diseases related to each system dysfunction, and decide for yourself which symptoms most affect your life and, as a consequence, what order of priority you wish to give to correcting any identified set of dysfunctions.

If necessary, you will also need to consult your doctor. If you have a number of disease diagnoses, then this is absolutely essential. Be prepared to spend time (and as a consequence, perhaps money) on a longer consultation with your doctor. Medical tests may also be in order to establish a present baseline for your health. Where issues of glycemic control, blood pressure or cholesterol levels are concerned, positive changes may already have happened as a result of work done during the preceding two phases. You may also need to discuss your medications and how they relate to any potential nutritional supplement interventions you are considering.

Note at this point you should only be addressing your highest priority health concern. Do not overdo your supplement program. This can be both expensive and unnecessary.

Often you will find that if you can work with the underlying primary health problem, secondary conditions will improve considerably as well. But if not, we can still work with these secondary dysfunctions in the near future (Phase 4, in four weeks).

Obviously this does not apply to prescription medicines, particularly if you are using multiple drugs for various conditions. **At no point should you change your prescription medicine without discussion and approval from your doctor.** As previously discussed, you may need to find a doctor willing to work with your desire to take an integrative approach to your health condition. This does not necessarily mean coming off all medicine.

Rather it implies finding a minimalist regime in which a minimum of prescription medication can be used to achieve effective change in combination with nutritional supplementation and lifestyle modification.

This is also the time to begin the Challenge Phase of the Food Elimination Regime. Ironically, many people feel so much better and/or have lost so much weight after three weeks on the Elimination Phase that they do not wish to reintroduce foods. If this is the case for you, resist the urge to continue on a restricted diet. The Elimination Phase is part of a process, not a diet on its own. For if you eliminate a considerable number of foods from your diet unnecessarily over the longer term, you risk nutritional deficiency from a lack of food variety.

During Phase 3 you should therefore focus upon:

1. Reviewing the chapter introduction questions in Section 5 as well as, if necessary, discussions with your doctor (where diagnosable disease or prescription medication usage exists). Decide what, if any, is the primary health dysfunction you wish to address. If you have not yet undertaken diagnostic testing of suspected or possible conditions (e.g. cholesterol, blood pressure, glucose tolerance test etc), now is the time to do so.

2. Begin to reintroduce foods withdrawn during the Elimination phase of the Food Elimination Regime, in order to establish whether or not you are intolerant to them.

3. Continue to commit to ongoing lifestyle modification activities as introduced during the first two Phases.

4. Re-read pertinent chapters to establish appropriate supplementation and other forms of specific interventions. Ensure that no contraindications exist preventing you from using the suggested intervention (you may need to discuss this with an appropriate doctor). If you have not committed to the Food Elimination Regime, apply yourself to this program for the following four weeks. Remember, however, that nutritional supplementation is usually necessary for a full three months, so do not stop supplementing when only halfway through a regime.

PHASE 4

Addressing Other Health Dysfunctions

Time Frame: As required
(usually in 3-month increments)

Hopefully, you have seen some progress in your wellbeing by this stage. You should have worked out whether or not you have Food Intolerances, and as a consequence have made short-term adjustments to the general Healthy Eating Plan recommended. Your main set of health symptoms as clustered about a particular health dysfunction have been addressed, which may be carrying improvements into other systems as well, due to the interrelationships within the whole Mindbody Being.

Excellent. Time for review and, if necessary, adaptation to your Whole Health Plan. Remembering that your ultimate goal, whether or not it is fully achievable, is a supplement free, medication free state dependent only on the fundamentals of natural health (exercise, diet, emotional management etc) to maintain a state of complete wellbeing.

And so to the crucial stage of review and adaptation that should occur **EVERY MONTH** until you are satisfied that you have covered all aspects of your health appropriately:

1. Review any health system you may already have addressed. Have you achieved a state of wellness and balance in this system in terms of your active interventions? If not, continue your present health intervention for a further month (maximum of three months), whether or not you institute any further actions for other health systems.

2. Look at any other set of signs and symptoms indicative of a system dysfunction. Simply do this by reviewing the questions at the start of the relevant chapters in Section 5. Are there any other systems you wish to address? If so, choose the problem of the highest priority to you (having hopefully discussed your list of priorities previously with your doctor).

3. Re-read the pertinent chapter for this issue to establish appropriate supplementation and other forms of intervention. Ensure that no contraindications exist which may prevent you from using the suggested intervention (you may need to discuss this with an appropriate doctor). If further supplementation has begun, it is likely that you will need to apply yourself to this addition to your program for the following three months.

4. Continue to reintroduce foods withdrawn during the Elimination Phase of the Food Elimination Regime, in order to establish whether or not you are intolerant to them. On completion of the Food Elimination Regime, finalise a Healthy Eating Plan with the initial exclusion of foods to which you are intolerant.

PUTTING IT ALL TOGETHER

PHASE 5

Weaning Supplementation

Time Frame: *As and when required*

If you have undertaken a supplement intervention program to alleviate a health dysfunction or disease, do you need to continue supplementing in the long-term?

The answer generally is no, although in some instances you might be unlucky enough to need ongoing treatment. The key question is, do you continue to need a higher dose of vitamin and mineral intake than you can achieve from your Healthy Eating Plan to stabilise your health state?

How do you work this out?

First of all, wait until you feel that the gains you have made in a particular area have stabilised. Ideally, this would be when you no longer have any symptoms of dysfunction or disease, however given the complex nature of health issues, this may instead be a plateau in the gains you will make from a supplement program, after which you may still need to rely on medication.

Next, diminish the dosage by a convenient amount, which will depend upon the dosage you are taking. For instance, if you were taking two tablets of a supplement to attain your dosage, you might now halve the dosage. The rate at which you wean should depend upon the extent of your previous symptoms and concerns. It is suggested you wean more slowly if you previously had more intense or serious dysfunction or disease.

Remain at your new dose for one to two weeks and monitor your symptoms. If your symptoms do not return, further reduce or even cease your dosage and again monitor for two weeks. Repeat as required to wean off your supplements, unless symptoms return.

If symptoms return, what do you do?

Again, this is simple. Return to the next highest dose in which you did not experience symptoms. And remain on this dose for a further period until you wish to try and wean again. There are some people (usually those with structural or genetically linked disorders) who find they need to continue on a low dose nutritional supplement in order to maintain a better state of wellbeing.

Note that if you have several different dysfunctions that you are sequentially addressing with a supplement program, then you can also wean different supplements at different times. For instance, if you start during Phase 3 with addressing heart health due to high cholesterol levels, and then decide to finetune your health by working on overcoming a low Immune System, you should wean your cholesterol lowering supplement programme after three months, but wean your Immune System Support regime a few weeks later. This sequential rather than simultaneous weaning of supplements is preferable from the perspective of understanding what is happening with your health, because it is easier to identify the supplement that is making the greatest difference. It is generally recommended, however, that only one (or maximum two) body systems be worked on simultaneously. Despite the very best intentions, too many supplements taken at once more often than not leads to an ultimate failure in compliance.

A further point to note is that many dysfunction or disease indicators rely on clinical tests rather than symptoms. Thus follow-up tests may be required to identify when a dysfunctional state or disease has been stabilised, and subsequently whether or not weaning is indicated. Cholesterol is such an example, as may be blood sugar levels (BSL's), insulin levels, urinary telopeptides (for osteoporosis) and so forth. Working with your naturopath, doctor or other health practitioner in such cases will therefore be essential in determining your progress and your success.

Can you remain on a supplement program to ensure that you maintain good health? That is entirely up to you. As long as you do not consume toxic levels of a supplement and have reviewed any possible interactions with medications, there are few other risks to worry about.

After all, this is the fundamental reasoning behind taking a multivitamin. Yet in effect your average multivitamin is an arbitrary choice of maintenance supplementation. Your first healthy supplement is, of course, having a Healthy Eating Plan. But you can achieve multivitamin insurance at any level depending upon your own willingness to finance the endeavour, and, indeed, your own need for higher individual doses as determined by your weaning process.

Your insurance dosage will start, if you have had a health dysfunction, at the level at which you find your health symptoms and dysfunctions no longer exist after the above weaning process. After all, this will represent your personal supplement needs for maintaining your present levels of health. After which, any top up in dosage is added protection for your future health needs (necessary or otherwise) as long as a level of toxicity is not reached.

Reducing your program applies to supplements only. There is no justification for weaning most other parts of this program; your Healthy Eating Plan, following the Pleasure and Passion principles, Exercise, Sleep Health and so forth. After all, these are fundamental principles of healthy living so they need to be pursued on an ongoing basis. The only exception is re-evaluating Food Intolerances, which will be discussed in Phase 7 of this plan.

Important Note:

Do not under any circumstances use the above approach to wean off any prescription medication. The above applies to nutritional supplements only. Prescription medication use should only ever be altered after advice from your prescribing doctor.

PHASE 6

Health Maintenance

The Health Maintenance Stage requires little explanation. Having now established Your Whole Health Program, it is time to commit to the long-term maintenance of your health. This means continuing to:

1. Develop a love of Self that puts Self health first as a priority in life.
2. Live according to the Passion and Pleasure Principles.
3. Improve Your Relationships.
4. Develop Emotional Intelligence.
5. Commit to Stress Reduction techniques.
6. Exercise Regularly.
7. Develop the ability to Relax.
8. Commit to Sleep Health.
9. Maintain your Healthy Eating Plan, individualised by an awareness of which foods to which you are presently intolerant.
10. Use Supplements if you have decided to continue a maintenance program of nutrients.

PUTTING IT ALL TOGETHER

PHASE 7

Health and Food Intolerance Reviews

As previously noted, we encourage you to establish regular Health Reviews to ensure you maintain your sense of wellbeing. An easy way to do this is to put a date in your diary every three months when you will review the health dysfunction questions from this book. This will ensure you will identify any emerging health dysfunctions as early as possible, and be able to respond to them effectively.

One particularly pertinent area to review is any Food Intolerance that you may have previously identified. For Food Intolerances are dynamic, and as your health state changes, so may the presence or absence of many Food Intolerances. Improve the health of your gastrointestinal system, reduce your stress levels, or change your medication and there is a chance that a Food Intolerance may be diminished (i.e. you may be able to consume a greater volume of a food than previously identified) or eradicated altogether. On the other hand, start to disrespect your health, and previously experienced or even new Food Intolerances may subsequently arise.

Therefore, if you have previously identified Food Intolerances it is suggested you review each food identified every three to six months to establish whether or not you remain intolerant. Optimistically, you may find on reintroduction that you are able to consume at least a limited volume of the food in question. To review a food you should:

1. Reintroduce only one food at a time.
2. Reintroduce your chosen food in a small volume only.
3. Establish whether or not previously experienced symptoms of Food Intolerance return at this volume of consumption.
4. Progressively increase the volume of the food you consume until you achieve a sensible serving size, as long as symptoms do not return.
5. If symptoms return, reduce your serving size to a volume you previously did not react to, and establish whether or not you can continue consuming this volume of food without experiencing symptoms.
6. Integrate your current knowledge of Food Tolerance and Intolerance into your revised Healthy Eating Plan.

Remember, the more diverse your diet, the healthier you are likely to be, given that you have minimised your Food Intolerances. Therefore the more regularly you review your Food Intolerances, the more likely it will be that you can diversify your diet, meanwhile enjoying all the succulent flavours on offer. Otherwise you may commit to an overly restrictive diet, risking nutrient deficiency and boredom over the long term.

Good luck, enjoy the journey and always remember to live your best life!

APPENDIX

Finding a Professional

It is essential that you establish a relationship with a person who has the knowledge, skills and integrity to honour your health, happiness and wellbeing. While no guarantee of this, the various registered professional bodies and associations for medical professionals allow some security in making this choice. In no way do we imply by the following list that unregistered professions or individuals do not have the skills to match your needs, but we strongly advise under all circumstances that you question your choice of any practitioner (registered or otherwise) until you feel comfortable with this choice.

All **medical doctors** are registered professionals, but if you are looking for a doctor with an interest in nutritional or complementary health areas there are two organisations with which they may be affiliated:

1) The Australasian Integrative Medical Association (AIMA). An association of doctors and other health professionals with a wide interest in integrating all medical approaches into integrated treatment approaches. **www.aima.net.au**

2) The Australasian College of Nutrition and Environmental Medicine (ACNEM). A training body for doctors who wish to forward their education in nutritional and environmental medicine. Doctors who are affiliated with ACNEM may identify that they do so as either a member (MACNEM) or fellow (FACNEM). **www.acnem.org**

Naturopathic/Nutritionist/Massage Therapists etc. Two main professional organisations exist to which complementary practitioners may be affiliated. They are:

1) Australian Traditional Medical Society (ATMS) **www.atms.com.au**
2) Australian Natural Therapists Association **www.anta.com.au**

The **pathology tests** recommended in this book, where not available from your local pathologist, may be accessed through either:

1) Metametrix Clinical Laboratories **www.metametrix.com.au**
2) Analytical Reference Laboratories **www.arlaus.com.au**
3) Path Lab **www.pathlab.com.au**

The following organisations are some of the professional bodies representing other appropriate **health practitioners:**

1) Australian Physiotherapy Association **www.physiotherapy.asn.au**
2) Chiropractor's Association of Australia **www.chiropractors.asn.au**
3) Australian Osteopathic Association
   www.osteopathy.com.au
4) Australian Psychological Society
   www.psychology.org.au

Other Titles from New Holland ...

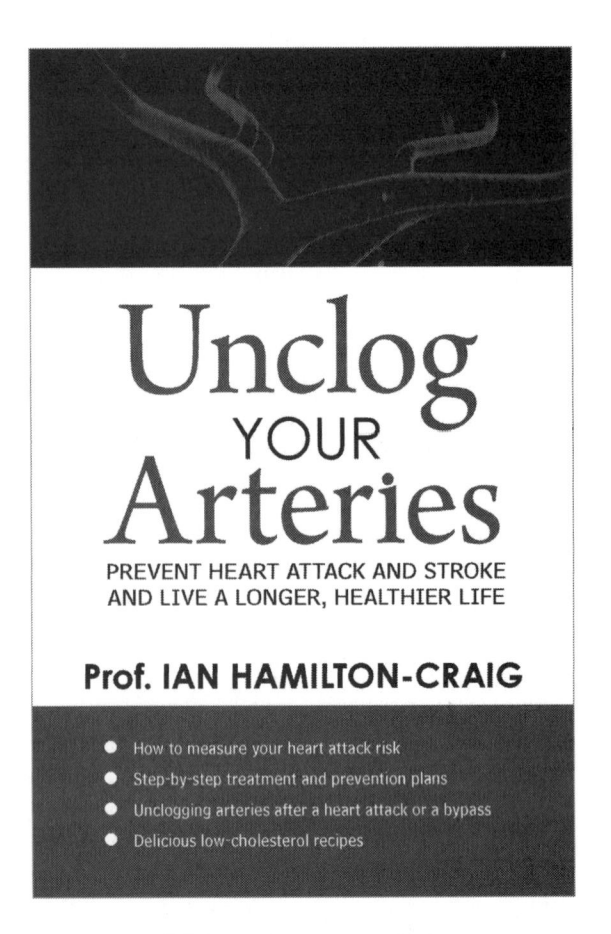

Unclog YOUR Arteries

PREVENT HEART ATTACK AND STROKE
AND LIVE A LONGER, HEALTHIER LIFE

Prof. IAN HAMILTON-CRAIG

- How to measure your heart attack risk
- Step-by-step treatment and prevention plans
- Unclogging arteries after a heart attack or a bypass
- Delicious low-cholesterol recipes

ISBN 9781741106039

NEW HOLLAND

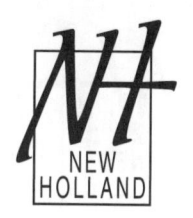

Heart Food
the Healthy Heart Cookbook

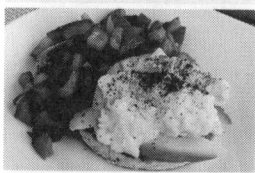

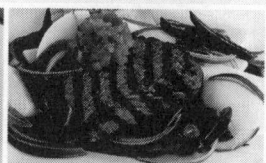

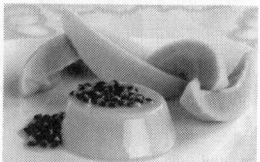

The proven way to protect your heart

- Eat well, lose weight and feel great
- Boost your energy and manage your blood glucose
- Over 80 delicious, easy-to-prepare recipes

Veronica Cuskelly
Nicole Senior

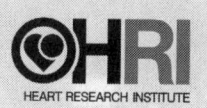

HRI HEART RESEARCH INSTITUTE

ISBN 9781741105957

NEW HOLLAND

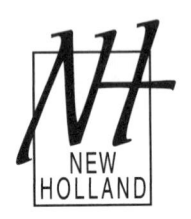

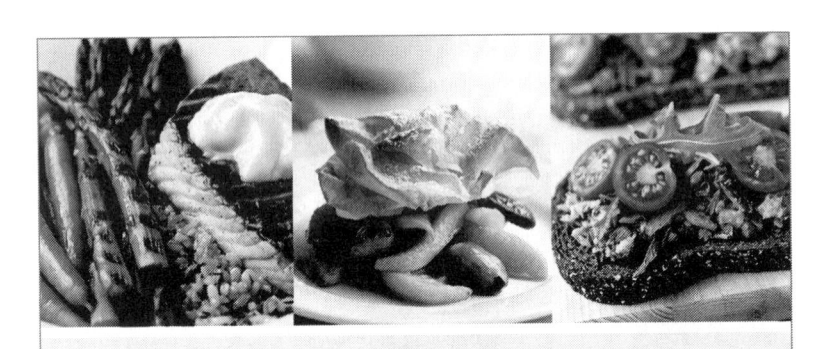

Eat to beat
cholesterol

- how to lower your cholesterol level
- eating plans to suit your lifestyle
- over 100 recipes
- shopping and cooking tips

Nicole Senior APD & Veronica Cuskelly

ISBN 9781741104493

NEW HOLLAND

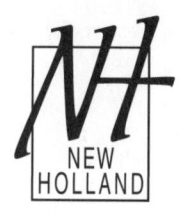

Asthma
Controlled Naturally
Techniques that Work

Natural therapies to help sufferers of asthma control their condition and become drug-free

Dr Ron Roberts
Chiropractor, Acupuncturist, Naturopath

ISBN 9781741105940